Paediatric and Neonatal Safe Transfer and Retrieval
The Practical Approach

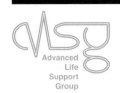

Paediatric and Neonatal Safe Transfer and Retrieval

The Practical Approach

Advanced Life Support Group

EDITED BY

Steve Byrne

Steve Fisher

Peter-Marc Fortune

Cassie Lawn

Sue Wieteska

WILEY-BLACKWELL

A John Wiley & Sons, Ltd., Publication

Library of Congress Cataloguing-in-Publication Data

Paediatric & neonatal safe transfer and retrieval : the practical approach / Advanced Life Support Group ; edited by Steve Byrne . . . [et al.].
    p. ; cm.
    "BMJ books."
    Includes bibliographical references and index.
    ISBN, 978-1-4051-6919-6 (alk. paper)
    1. Interhospital transport of children–Great Britain. 2. Pediatric emergency services–Great Britain. 3. Neonatal intensive care–Great Britain. I. Byrne, Steve, Dr. II. Advanced Life Support Group (Manchester, England) III. Title: Paediatric and neonatal safe transfer and retrieval.
    [DNLM: 1. Patient Transfer–organization & administration. 2. Transportation of Patients–organization & administration. 3. Child. 4. Critical Care–methods. 5. Infant. 6. Patient Care Team. WX 158 P126 2008]
    RA996.G7P43 2008
    362.198'9200941–dc22

                                                                                    2007047270

ISBN: 978-1-4051-6919-6

A catalogue record for this book is available from the British Library.

Set in 10 on 13 pt Meridien by SNP Best-set Typesetter Ltd., Hong Kong
Printed in Spain by GraphyCems, Navarra

1 2008

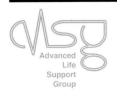

Contents

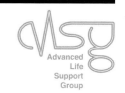

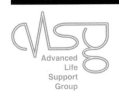

Advanced
Life
Support
Group

Working group

Neil Aiton NICU, *Brighton*

Peter Barry PICU, *Leicester*

Steve Byrne NICU, *Middlesbrough*

Ian Dady NICU, *Manchester*

Alan Fenton NICU, *Newcastle*

Steve Fisher ALSG, *Manchester*

Peter-Marc Fortune PICU, *Manchester*

Claire Harness Neonatology Transport, *Leeds*

Carol Jackson Neonatal Transport, *Liverpool*

Debbie Kenny Midwifery, University of Central Lancashire, *Preston*

Cassie Lawn NICU, *Brighton*

Andy Leslie Neonatology Transport, *Nottingham*

John Madar NICU, *Plymouth*

Dawn McKimm Paediatric Transport, *Belfast*

David Rowney Paediatric Anaesthesia and Intensive Care, *Edinburgh*

Sue Wieteska ALSG, *Manchester*

Contributors

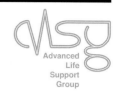

Steve Byrne Paediatrics/Neonatology, *Middlesbrough*

Ian Dady Neonatology, *Manchester*

Peter-Marc Fortune PICU, *Manchester*

Stephen Graham Anaesthetics, *Middlesbrough*

Carol Jackson Neonatal Transport, *Liverpool*

Cassie Lawn Neonatology, *Brighton*

Daniel Lutman Children's Acute Transport Service, *London*

John Madar Neonatology, *Plymouth*

Dawn McKimm Paediatric Transport Co-ordinator, *Belfast*

Mary Montgomery Children's Acute Transport Service, *London*

Kate Parkins PICU, *Liverpool*

Fiona Reynolds PICU, *Birmingham*

Michael Tremlett Anaesthetics, *Middlesbrough*

Allan Wardhaugh PICU, *Cardiff*

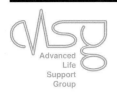

Preface

Over the last few years there has been a trend towards increased centralisation of secondary and tertiary paediatric services. A number of strong drivers lie behind this: the increasing complexity of the techniques available to support children when they are unwell, the need for expertise to be maintained in delivering such care to relatively low numbers of patients, and an ever increasing public expectation of what should be treated rather than palliated.

As a consequence of these demands there are now well over 10 000 interhospital transfers of unwell children and neonates every year in the UK. Most areas have specialised retrieval teams who will undertake these transfers wherever possible. However at the current time the transport service provision is both fragmented and heterogeneous in terms of the resources available. There are also a small proportion of children who, by virtue of their pathology, cannot wait for an offsite retrieval team to mobilise and undertake their transfer. Therefore it is not uncommon that non-specialist teams have to be mobilised by receiving hospitals to move their charges into receiving tertiary centres.

This book (and the associated course) has been developed to provide an introduction to the knowledge necessary to undertake the transfer of sick children and neonates. It is aimed both at those embarking on training in paediatric and neonatal transport and at those who might expect that they will have to undertake such transfers on an occasional basis. Although the focus is on interhospital transfers, the principles are also directly applicable every time a child is moved between clinical areas. There are inevitable discussions of clinical situations throughout the text; however, the focus is primarily on the logistics of the transfer process. Those whose primary requirement is to enhance their knowledge of resuscitation should direct their reading to the APLS and NLS textbooks and courses.

Paediatric and Neonatal Safe Transfer and Retrieval: The Practical Approach has been developed by a multiprofessional group from across the UK. A systematic approach is employed throughout that has been adapted from that used in the adult STaR course.

The book is divided into six parts. Part I provides an overview of the current delivery of children's transport services and introduces the ACCEPT approach that is utilised throughout the text. Part II examines the component parts of ACCEPT in detail. The practical issues that are encountered during the transfer process from an equipment perspective, and from a clinical perspective, are discussed in Parts III and IV, respectively. Part V discusses particular situations and provides additional background information that is required to plan for special circumstances. The appendices in Part VI contain supporting information and provide sample checklists and example documentation for those undertaking transfers.

Steve Byrne, Steve Fisher, Peter-Marc Fortune,
Cassie Lawn, Sue Wieteska

Acknowledgements

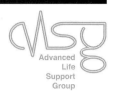

A great many people have worked hard to produce this book and the accompanying course. The editors would like to thank all the contributors for their efforts and all PaNSTaR (formally known as PNeoSTaR) providers and instructors who took the time to send their comments during the development of the text and the course.

The editors and ALSG would like to thank Neil Aiton, whose enthusiasm has driven this course forward.

Also, they would like to thank Carol Jackson, Elaine Metcalfe and Dawn McKimm for their contribution to the editing of Part II of the book.

We would also like to acknowledge and thank Helen Carruthers, MMAA and Kate Wieteska for producing the excellent line drawings that illustrate the text.

To maintain consistency between ALSG courses PaNSTaR has been closely linked to STaR (Safe Transfer and Retrieval). The PaNSTaR working group would like to acknowledge that a number of chapters in this book are based on *Safe Transfer and Retrieval: The Practical Approach*, 2nd edition and the PaNSTaR editors would like to thank all the people involved with the second edition of STaR: in particular, Pete Driscoll, Kevin Mackway-Jones, Elaine Metcalfe and Peter Oakley, and with special thanks to Ian Macartney.

Finally, we would like to thank, in advance, those of you who will attend the PaNSTaR course; no doubt you will have much constructive criticism to offer.

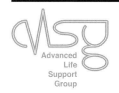
Advanced
Life
Support
Group

Contact details and website information

ALSG: www.alsg.org
BestBETS: www.bestbets.org

For details on ALSG courses visit the website or contact:
Advanced Life Support Group
ALSG Centre for Training and Development
29–31 Ellesmere Street
Swinton, Manchester M27 0LA
Tel: +44 (0) 161 794 1999
Fax: +44 (0) 161 794 9111
Email: enquiries@alsg.org

UPDATES

The material contained within this book is updated on a 4-yearly cycle. However, practice may change in the interim period. We will post any changes on the ALSG website, so we advise you to visit the website regularly to check for updates (www.alsg.org – click on updates). The website will provide you with a new page to download and replace the existing page in your book.

REFERENCES

To access references visit the ALSG website www.alsg.org – click on references.

TRANSFER SCENARIO BANK

This is a bank of worked 'real life' scenarios using the ACCEPT approach. This is an interactive site allowing sharing of transfer experiences and will be available via the ALSG website.

ON-LINE FEEDBACK

It is important to ALSG that the contact with our providers continues after a course is completed. We now contact everyone 6 months after their course has taken place, asking for on-line feedback on the course. This information is then used whenever the course is updated to ensure that the course provides optimum training for its participants.

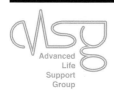

PART I
Introduction

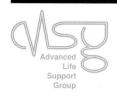

CHAPTER 1

Introduction

LEARNING OBJECTIVES

In this chapter you will learn about:
- Why unwell children are transferred between hospitals
- The issues that may adversely affect delivery of care

BACKGROUND

In children's critical care alone there are in excess of 5500 neonatal intensive care unit (NICU) and 5000 paediatric ICU (PICU) transfers between hospitals in the UK every year. In addition to this, there are numerous HDU (high dependency unit) and non-urgent transfers between centres and countless thousands of intrahospital transfers undertaken by healthcare professionals every year. Each one of these transfers represents an episode of care that is associated with a period of increased risk for both the child and the clinical staff. These risks can at best be eliminated and at least be minimised through appropriate training.

The PaNSTaR manual, with its associated course, is aimed at a multidisciplinary audience and has been developed to provide a comprehensive introduction and overview of the process of transferring unwell neonates, infants and children. Its conception followed from the success of the adult STaR manual and course. The underpinning concepts, and in particular the ACCEPT principles, described herein, are essentially the same. However the practicalities of transferring unwell children are significantly different. It is an old adage, but in this area perhaps never more true – children are not small adults!

Throughout the text 'child' or 'children' should be taken to refer to the entire age range (neonate up to 16 years of age). Where appropriate more specific references to particular age groups will be made where practices vary according to age. 'Neonates' is used to refer to all preterm babies and also term babies who are less than 28 days old. 'Infants' refers to all those under 1 year. Parent refers to any person with parental responsibility.

In addition to the practical differences associated with transferring children, there has also been a cultural change that has occurred, in many centres, of

---

Paediatric and Neonatal Safe Transfer and Retrieval: The Practical Approach, Edited by Steve Byrne, Steve Fisher, Peter-Marc Fortune, Cassie Lawn and Sue Wieteska. © 2008 Blackwell Publishing, ISBN: 978-1-4051-6919-6.

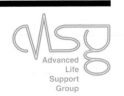

non-paediatricians distancing themselves from paediatric practice, triggered by the centralisation of paediatric services. Many district general hospital (DGH) practitioners, faced with a critically ill child, may now find themselves practising at the edge of their comfort zone. This is perhaps particularly true if they have to undertake a transfer.

Most NICUs and PICUs will have an associated retrieval team. However, most, if not all, of these teams are not sufficiently resourced to be able to provide a robust service 100% of the time. There will also be occasions, such as children with surgically treatable lesions after a traumatic head injury, where current practice would dictate that the referring hospital should undertake the transfer in order to minimise the time to the start of neurosurgery. At the current time these factors mean that referring centres may expect to carry out the transfer for between 25 and 30% of the children whom they refer for urgent tertiary care.

We anticipate that reading this manual and attending a PaNSTaR course will provide you with the basic strategies and background that you need to join a paediatric transfer team. It is important to note that proficiency in this area comes only with the additional training and experience that may be gained from working with practitioners already experienced in this area.

THE APPROACH TO TRANSFER

Any transfer process may be broken down into three components:
1 The organisational and management strategy
2 The practical issues
3 The training required for appropriate use of the equipment on the transfer.

The course focus is on the transportation of children between hospitals. However, the same approach can, and should, be applied to the transportation of unwell children within hospitals.

The usual purpose of an interhospital transfer or retrieval is either to allow the patient to be treated more effectively or to obtain additional diagnostic information, in a geographically separate site. Transfer in itself does not constitute therapy and represents a time of increased risk. It is therefore essential always to consider the risks versus the benefits before undertaking a potentially hazardous journey.

In the neonatal population babies may be transferred acutely because they require ICU therapy that is not available at the referring NICU or SCBU (special care baby unit). There are also a significant number of neonates who may be moved for specialist examinations or opinions. Infants and older children are primarily transferred when they are acutely unwell to a central PICU or HDU. Some transfers will also occur for secondary or tertiary opinions, but most of these patients will not present a significant clinical risk and will be transported by their parents. In all the acute cases children may sometimes have to be transferred significant distances, especially at busy times such as midwinter, because beds may not be available in their nearest tertiary centre.

Box 1.1 details the wide spectrum of clinical presentations that may be encountered. Diagnostic groups are in order, from most common to least common, based on Paediatric Intensive Care Audit Network (PICANET) data. Within the groups the top specific diagnoses are similarly listed.

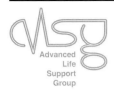

Box 1.1 Clinical conditions requiring transfer

Neonates
- Extreme prematurity
- Hyaline membrane disease
- Congenital abnormalities:
  - cardiac
  - respiratory
  - surgical
- Hypoxic ischaemic encephalopathy
- Meconium aspiration syndrome

Children
- Cardiovascular:
  - ventricular septal defect
  - tetralogy of Fallot
  - transposition of the great arteries
- Respiratory:
  - bronchiolitis
  - pneumonia
  - respiratory failure secondary to chronic or acute neurological conditions
  - status asthmaticus
- Neurological: status epilepticus (usually respiratory failure secondary to treatment)
- Gastrointestinal
- Infection:
  - sepsis (non-specified)
  - meningococcal sepsis
- Trauma:
  - traumatic head injury
  - burns
- Haematological/Oncological
- Postoperative
- Metabolic:
  - DKA (diabetic ketoacidosis)
  - inborn errors of metabolism
- Substance abuse/poisoning/overdose
- Liver failure

The source of these patients also varies widely:
- Delivery suite
- Emergency department
- NICUs
- Adult ICUs
- Paediatric wards
- Operating theatres
- HDUs
- CCUs (critical care units).

Emergency departments are probably the most frequent starting place for the movement of PICU patients. Sometimes children are moved to local critical care facilities before transfer. Either way the adequacy of resuscitation and the degree of packaging that will have been undertaken, before the arrival of the transfer team, is highly variable. When dispatching a team to undertake this task it is

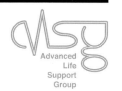

always best to assume they will need to do everything and therefore must have the knowledge and skills to do so.

Transfers are not infrequently associated with adverse events, which may be recorded on transfer forms. Those seen most commonly are:

- No capnography available (when clinically indicated)
- Equipment failure
- Significant hypotension
- Significant hypoxia
- Inadequate resuscitation
- Significant tachycardia
- Mechanical ventilator not available
- Delay in getting ambulance
- Ambulance getting lost en route
- Cardiac arrest in ambulance.

The number of interhospital transfers continues to rise. This is perhaps stimulated by an increasing expectation on the part of both the general public and healthcare professionals.

SUMMARY

The course and this manual provides those who may be involved with the transfer of unwell children with a systematic approach to guide their work. It does not seek to teach or develop the clinical skills required to undertake such care but it does provide a structure that should help eliminate most of the non-clinical pit-falls. At the end of the day, there is no substitute for clinical experience, which may be gained by working with those experienced in this field.

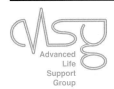

CHAPTER 2

The structured approach to transfers

LEARNING OBJECTIVES

In this chapter you will learn about:
- The principles of the safe transfer or retrieval of critically ill children
- The systematic ACCEPT approach for managing such children

INTRODUCTION

The aim of a safe transfer policy is to ensure that child care is streamlined and of the highest standard. To achieve this, the *right* child has to be taken at the *right* time, by the *right* people, to the *right* place by the *right* form of transport, and receive the *right* care throughout. This requires a systematic approach that incorporates a high level of planning and preparation before the child is moved. One such approach is the ACCEPT method (Box 2.1), which is used in adults, it may also be used for paediatrics and neonates (Figure 2.1).

Box 2.1 The systematic approach to transfer of a child

A   Assessment
C   Control
C   Communication
E   Evaluation
P   Preparation and packaging
T   Transportation

Following ACCEPT ensures that appropriate assessments and procedures are carried out. This method also correctly emphasises the preparation that is required before the child is transported. The component parts of ACCEPT are outlined below. Subsequent chapters deal with each part in detail.

Paediatric and Neonatal Safe Transfer and Retrieval: The Practical Approach, Edited by Steve Byrne, Steve Fisher, Peter-Marc Fortune, Cassie Lawn and Sue Wieteska. © 2008 Blackwell Publishing, ISBN: 978-1-4051-6919-6.

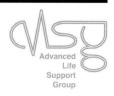

ACCEPT Model
Retrieval team does transfer

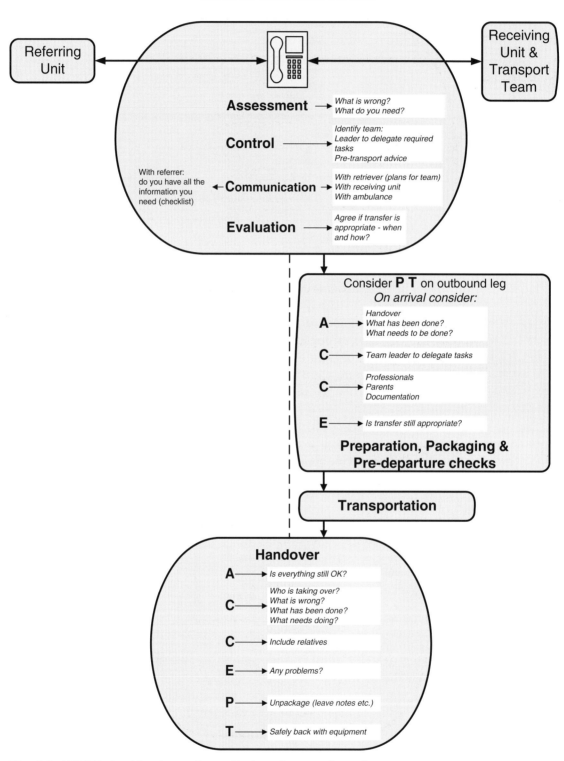

Fig. 2.1 ACCEPT algorithm for use in paediatric and neonatal transfers.

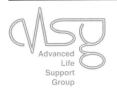

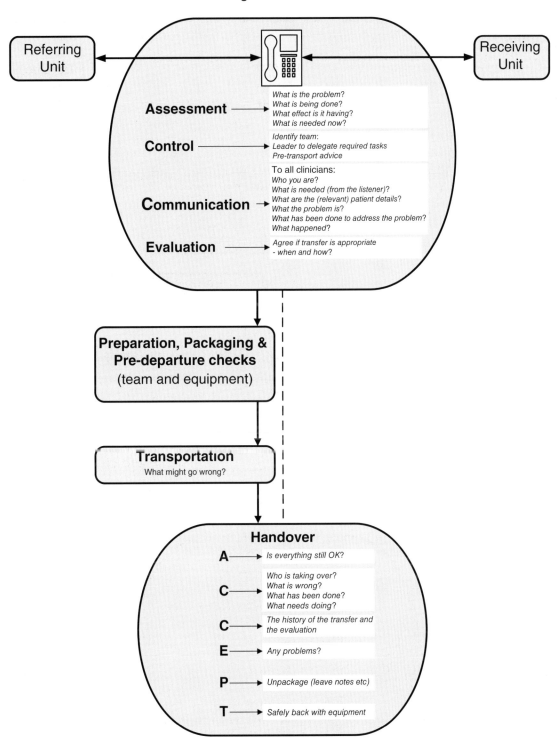

Fig. 2.1 (*Continued*)

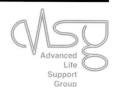

ASSESSMENT

The first thing to do is assess the situation. Sometimes the clinician involved in the transportation has also been involved in the care given up to that point. Increasingly, however, the transporter will have been brought in specifically for that purpose and will have no prior knowledge of the child's clinical history.

CONTROL

Once assessment is complete, the transport organiser needs to take control of the situation. This requires:
- Identification of the clinical team leader
- Identification of the tasks to be carried out
- Allocation of tasks to individuals or teams.

The lines of responsibility must be established promptly. In theory, ultimate responsibility is held jointly by the referring consultant clinician, the receiving consultant clinician and the transfer personnel at different stages of the transfer process. There should always be a named person with overall responsibility for organising the transfer.

COMMUNICATION

Moving ill children from one place to another obviously requires cooperation and the involvement of many people. Therefore key personnel need to be informed when transportation is being considered (Box 2.2). Communication may take a long time to complete if one person does it all. It is therefore advisable to share the tasks between appropriate people, taking into account expertise and local policies. In all cases it is important that information is passed on clearly and unambiguously. This is particularly the case when talking to people over the telephone. It is useful to plan what to say before telephoning and to use the systematic summary shown in Box 2.3. It is also useful in complex conversations to summarise the situation and repeat what you need from the listener at the end.

Box 2.2 People who need to know about a transfer

Current (local) clinical team:
- Consultant in charge
- Clinicians at bedside
- Referring doctor/nurse
- Lead nurse

Transfer team:
- Transfer coordinator should disperse information to:
  Consultant in charge
  Clinician(s) undertaking transfer
  Ambulance providers

Receiving team:
- Transfer coordinator or receiving unit coordinator disperses information to:
  Consultant in charge
  Receiving doctors
  Receiving nursing staff

The child's relatives

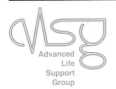

> **Box 2.3 Key elements in any communication**
>
> - Who you are
> - What is needed (from the listener)
> - What are the (relevant) child's details
> - What the problem is
> - What has been done to address the problem
> - What happened
> - What is needed from the listener

The responses to all these questions should be documented in the child's notes. The person in overall charge can then assimilate this information so that a proper evaluation of the child's requirements for transportation can be made.

EVALUATION

The aim of evaluation is to assess whether transfer is appropriate for the child and, if so, what is the clinical urgency? Whilst evaluation is a dynamic process which starts from first contact with the child, it is usually only when the first phase of ACCEPT (that is, ACC) has been completed that enough information will have been gathered to fully evaluate the transfer needs.

Is transfer appropriate for this child?

Critically ill babies and children require transfer because of the need for:
- Specialist treatment
- Specialist investigations unavailable in the referring hospital
- Specialist facilities unavailable in the referring hospital.

The risks involved in transfer must be balanced against the risks of staying and the benefits of care that can be given only by the receiving unit.

What clinical urgency does this child have?

Once it has been established that transfer is needed, the urgency must be evaluated. The degree of urgency for transfer and the severity of illness may be used to rank the child's transfer needs (Box 2.4). This hierarchy also helps determine both the personnel required and the mode of transport.

> **Box 2.4 Transfer categories**
>
> - Emergency – time critical: stable/unstable
> - Urgent: stable/unstable
> - Non-urgent (elective)

PREPARATION AND PACKAGING

Both preparation and packaging have the aim of ensuring that transport proceeds uneventfully and with no deterioration in the child's condition. The first stage (preparation) involves completion of stabilisation and preparation of transfer team personnel and equipment. The second stage (packaging) involves the final measures that need to be taken to ensure the security and safety of the child, equipment and staff during the transportation itself.

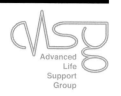

Child preparation

To reduce complications during any journey, meticulous resuscitation and stabilisation should be carried out before transfer. This may involve carrying out procedures requested by the receiving hospital or unit. The standard airway, breathing and circulation (ABC) approach should be followed. The airway must be cleared and secured and appropriate respiratory support established.

Venous access is essential and should preferably include a minimum of two cannulae or a sutured multi-lumen central line. The child must have received adequate fluid resuscitation to ensure optimal tissue oxygenation. Hypovolaemic children tolerate the inertial forces of transportation very poorly.

Occasionally, in time-critical situations such as an expanding intracranial lesion requiring neurosurgery, this process may not be fully completed before packing and transport. Decisions to transfer in those circumstances should be taken only by senior personnel.

> Inadequate resuscitation or missed illnesses (and injuries) may result in instability during transfer and may adversely affect the child's outcome.

Equipment preparation

All equipment must be tested and have adequate power reserves. Supplies of drugs and fluids should be more than adequate for the whole of the intended journey. Particular care should be taken with supplies of oxygen, inotropes, sedative drugs and batteries for portable electronic equipment. A member of the team should be allocated the task of ensuring that all the child's documents, including case notes, investigations, radiographs, reports and a transfer form, accompany the child.

The team should carry a mobile phone together with contact names and numbers to enable direct communication with both the receiving and base units. In addition, all personnel need appropriate clothing, food if the journey is long, and enough money to enable them to get home independently if needed.

Personnel preparation

The number and nature of staff accompanying children during transport will depend on their transfer category.

All staff must practise within their competences. Whatever the category of the child, all personnel should be familiar with the relevant transfer procedures and the equipment that is to be used, as well as the details of the child's clinical condition. The team should carry accident insurance with adequate provision for personal injury or death sustained during the transfer.

Packaging

All lines and drains must be secured to the child, the child must be secured to the trolley and the trolley must be secured to the transport vehicle. This is especially important in neonatal transfers using a transport system that typically weighs over 100 kg. In an ambulance all equipment fastenings should be CEN compliant.

Chest drains should be secured and unclamped, with any underwater seal device replaced by an appropriate flutter valve system. A special kit should be prepared to enable chest drain insertion or replacement en route if necessary.

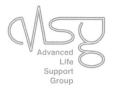

The child should be adequately covered to prevent heat loss. Care must be taken to ensure that coverings are arranged to permit ready access to the child, lines and drains during transfer.

TRANSPORTATION

Mode of transport

The choice of transport needs to take into account several factors (Box 2.5).

Box 2.5 Factors affecting mode of transfer

- Nature of illness
- Urgency of transfer
- Mobilisation time
- Geographical factors
- Weather
- Traffic conditions
- Cost

Road ambulances are by far the most common means of transport used in the UK. They have a low overall cost and rapid mobilisation time, and are not generally affected by weather conditions. They also give rise to less physiological disturbance.

Air transfer may be preferred for journeys of more than 50 miles (80 km) or 2 hours in duration, or if road access is difficult. The speed of the journey itself has to be balanced against organisational delays and also the need for inter-vehicle transfer at the start and end of the journey. Staff undertaking air transfers should have received specific training with regard to safety and flight physiology. They should not undertake such transfers without supervised experience.

Care during transport

Destabilisation may occur during transportation and may arise from the effects of the transport environment on the vulnerable physiology of the child. Careful preparation can minimise the deleterious effects of inertial forces, such as tipping, acceleration and deceleration, as well as changes in temperature and barometric pressure.

The standard of care and the level of monitoring carried out before transfer needs to be continued, as far as possible, during the transfer. Monitoring should include oxygen saturation, ECG and direct arterial pressure monitoring in most children. End-tidal carbon dioxide ($ETCO_2$) monitoring should be used in all intubated children (and increasingly neonates).

The child should be well covered and kept warm during the transfer. Road speed decisions depend on clinical urgency. Although blue lights and sirens may be appropriate in order to get through heavy traffic, excessive speed is very rarely indicated. It is a risk to the child, the transfer team and the general public, and should be the exception rather than the rule.

With adequate preparation, the transportation phase is usually incident free. However, untoward events do occur. Should this be the case, the child needs to be reassessed using the ABC approach and appropriate corrective measures then instituted. If the transport team need to release their seatbelts, the ambulance must slow down immediately, and then stop at the first available safe place. If a major deterioration occurs, transfer to the nearest hospital for further stabilisation and support may be appropriate. The benefits of intervention should always be weighed against the risks of delaying arrival at the receiving hospital with its better facilities. Following any untoward events, communications with the receiving unit are important. This should follow the systematic summary described earlier.

Handover

At the end of the transfer direct contact with the receiving team must be established. A succinct, systematic summary of the child and transfer must be provided before transferring the child on to the local bed/cot, monitoring and ventilator. It must be accompanied by a written record of the child's history, vital signs, therapy and significant clinical events during transfer. All the other documents that have been taken with the child should also be handed over. Once verbal handover has been completed the child may be moved from the transport trolley to the receiving unit's cot or bed.

The team can then retrieve all their equipment and personnel and make their way back to their home unit.

SUMMARY

The safe transfer and retrieval of a child requires a systematic approach. The ACCEPT method ensures that all essential components of the transfer process are included.

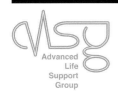
Advanced
Life
Support
Group

PART II
Managing the transfer

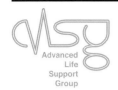

CHAPTER 3

Assessment and control

LEARNING OBJECTIVES

In this chapter you will learn about:
- A systematic approach to assessing a potential transfer situation
- The steps necessary to control the situation

INTRODUCTION

A clinician involved in a potential transfer situation may have had no contact with the child before receiving a phone call from a member of the treating clinical team. It is important to learn how to assess such a situation quickly and effectively. This must be done before management of the child continues.

Proper assessment requires consideration of both the child's condition and the actions and competences of the transferring team. The answers to several key questions will help this process (Box 3.1).

Box 3.1 Assessment questions

- What is the problem?
- What is being done?
- What effect is it having?
- What is needed now?

ASSESSING THE SITUATION

After a careful enquiry into the history of the current illness or injury, an ABCDE approach should be adopted to identify the immediate and predictable clinical needs of the child. The question 'What is being done?' provides the opportunity

Paediatric and Neonatal Safe Transfer and Retrieval: The Practical Approach, Edited by Steve Byrne, Steve Fisher, Peter-Marc Fortune, Cassie Lawn and Sue Wieteska. © 2008 Blackwell Publishing, ISBN: 978-1-4051-6919-6.

to check that appropriate treatment, if not already being undertaken on arrival, is started. This question also reflects 'What should be done?' The effect of clinical interventions should be the subject of continuous evaluation: Is what is being done working? If not, what is needed to improve the situation? With appropriate resuscitative measures the child will usually be stabilised for transfer. What is then needed is a safe transfer to a ward or department for definitive care.

Communications should start with a summary of the problem; in some cases this may be easy to describe succinctly. Often, however, children have a complex medical history, and it is difficult to rationalise all the available data into a presentable and reproducible format. During the transfer process the 'problem' may have to be communicated to a number of people in a short space of time. Health service professionals are not usually tolerant of long-winded explanations. As we live in a world of 'sound bites', a useful technique is to learn to reduce a complicated story into a sound bite of one short sentence – an easily repeatable description of the most relevant aspects of the case. After this sound bite introduction, a quick ABCDE description of what has been done, and the effect, should continue with the request for transfer to a particular ward or department.

CONTROLLING THE SITUATION

Following the initial assessment, someone needs to take control of the situation. This involves:
- Identifying the team leader
- Identifying the tasks to be carried out
- Allocating tasks to individuals or teams.

Identifying the team leader
The transfer team leader will be in overall control of the transfer – this person will have responsibility for ensuring that the child's clinical care continues, while others are directed to deal with communications, organise resources and timing, carry out the evaluation, oversee packaging and initiate the transfer itself.

The team leader may be in charge of the clinical care of the child. If he or she is not, then close liaison with the clinical team leader is essential.

As well as being present, the transfer team leader must be experienced enough to be capable of successfully seeing the task through and be sufficiently senior to have the confidence of their peers. In any given situation, an appropriate leader is usually obvious, because of either their experience or seniority. If this is not the case the most experienced member of staff present should take this role initially, while seeking senior or experienced help. Appropriate support should also be offered to those in training who may take on this role under the supervision of a suitable trainer. Usual communications in this instance should be directed to the trainee not the trainer.

Task identification
Once control has been established, clinical care of the child must continue; communication with those who need to know then becomes a priority. Resources including staffing, equipment and drugs will need to be identified and located. This can be summarised in a general task list, which will obviously have to be expanded and developed for individual clinical situations (Box 3.2).

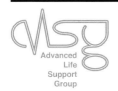

> **Box 3.2 General task list**
>
> • Direct clinical care
> • Communications
> • Assemble required equipment and resources

Task allocation

Tasks should be allocated by the transfer team leader. Competence is key and tasks should be given only to staff who have the appropriate training and expertise. The team leader will need to consider the relative priority of each task and the scope for concurrent activity.

SUMMARY

The first step for the team leader is to assess the situation, determine what treatment is ongoing, its effect and what else is required. To carry this out the team leader needs to take control of the situation by allocating key roles to staff.

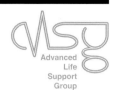

CHAPTER 4

Communication

LEARNING OBJECTIVES

In this chapter you will learn about:
- Who should communicate and who should be communicated with during the transfer process
- What needs to be communicated during the transfer process

INTRODUCTION

As already stated in Chapter 2, the successful transfer of an ill patient from one clinical area to another requires the coordinated effort of individuals from a number of different teams. Good communication is essential to achieve this required cooperation and coordination. It is for this reason that communication is in a pivotal position in the ACCEPT approach.

Communication begins, on an individual level, as soon as the initial referral has been received. The responsible clinician must communicate effectively with those who are already dealing with the child, so that an accurate assessment can be carried out. Good communication must then be continued through the control phase to the point when the decision to transfer has been made. At this point the agreed need for transfer must be communicated to those who need to know. Ideally the receiving clinical area will have been identified and have agreed to accept the child. However, in some regions the transport team will be mobilised in advance of an allocation from the receiving unit.

Once the transfer is under way, good communication remains an essential part of the process. Both referring and receiving teams must be kept informed, as must the transport providers. Relatives and supporting services should be kept up to date at all stages of the transfer and written records must be kept.

Many different methods of communication will be necessary during the transfer. Initially (at the referring unit) most of the communication will be face to face or by phone. Once transport is under way mobile phones and radios may be used. Finally, face-to-face communication with the receiving team will be important, as will the delivery of an accurate written record.

Paediatric and Neonatal Safe Transfer and Retrieval: The Practical Approach, Edited by Steve Byrne, Steve Fisher, Peter-Marc Fortune, Cassie Lawn and Sue Wieteska. © 2008 Blackwell Publishing, ISBN: 978-1-4051-6919-6.

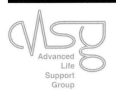

WHO COMMUNICATES WITH WHOM?

The clinician responsible for the decision to transfer the child has the ultimate responsibility for co-ordinating communication that occurs both within the referring unit and between this unit and outside agencies. Similarly, the accepting clinician in the receiving unit has ultimate responsibility for co-ordinating communication at that end of the transfer chain. Both these clinicians may have to delegate some of these calls to other members of staff. However, key calls, such as those offering and accepting the child should normally be between these two. A list of some of the calls that may be necessary during the transfer process is given in Table 4.1 together with a list of appropriate staff who could be asked to make them.

Table 4.1 Calls made during transfer

	Nature	Responsibility
Transfer calls	Seek availability of bed	Clinician or administrator
	Book transfer	Clinician or administrator
	Advise receiving unit	Clinician
	Arrange staff:	
	Nursing	Nurse
	Ambulance	Clinician or administrator
	Medical	Doctor/transport practitioner
Clinical calls	Discuss with specialist	Doctor/transport practitioner
	Negotiate bed	Clinician
Information calls	Inform responsible consultants	Doctor/transport practitioner
	Inform relatives	Clinician

Even if calls are delegated, it is important that the outcome be reported to the responsible clinicians at each unit, so that they maintain an overview of the transfer as it occurs.

WHAT NEEDS TO BE COMMUNICATED?

Successful communication has occurred when all the necessary information has been passed on and understood by all the relevant people. During the transfer process, it can be seen that successful communication requires both clinical and logistical arrangements to be made and understood. As already noted, each case communication should consist of the following:
- Who you are
- What is needed (from the listener)
- What the (relevant) child's details are
- What the problem is
- What has been done to address the problem
- What happened
- What is needed (from the listener)

Who you are
Not only should the instigators of the call identify who they are, they should also state whether they are calling on their own behalf or have been assigned the task of communication by someone else. This ensures that the receiver of the call has

a clear idea as to whether the call has been instigated at an appropriate level, and helps to avoid misunderstandings later on. Sometimes the most senior clinician will be actively involved with the child's intensive care and may need to delegate the call to a more junior team member.

What is needed (from the listener)

This is the most important part of the call from the perspective of both the caller and the listener. It is therefore essential that the need be stated clearly and succinctly. To ensure that this is the case, a little time to plan your essential requirements from the listener will be beneficial before the call is initiated.

What the (relevant) child's details are

The exact details that are relevant will vary. However, a minimum dataset consists of the following:

- Child's full name
- Child's date of birth or age
- Current location.

Many receiving units have proformas (Appendix D) for collecting the necessary information. If these are available to the referring units, it allows them to gather the relevant information systematically. Regionalised proformas are ideal.

What the problem is

This builds upon what you have already requested from the listener. Communications designed to book an intensive care bed will be very different from those for an ambulance service to arrange transportation. In the first example, considerable clinical information may be required, and the exact amount will be a matter of negotiation between the instigator and the receiver of the call. This negotiation is an important aspect of the call: the instigator should prepare a concise verbal presentation of the clinical details, including current vital signs and laboratory results. He or she should also ensure that the receiving unit is informed about any other potentially relevant details about the child, such as history of prematurity, previous ICU admissions or a known cardiac defect. It is helpful to have other potentially useful information to hand as well.

Much time is wasted during telephone referrals when every request for additional information is followed by a need for further communication with a third party in the background; the need for this can be reduced by the availability of a completed proforma.

What has been done to address the problem and what happened

When making a referral for ongoing clinical care, the treatment given so far, and the response to that treatment will be very important to the recipient of the call. They will need to assure themselves that all appropriate measures have been undertaken to ensure that the child's care is optimised and the transfer is appropriate. For example:

- What has been done? Use an ABCDE approach
- What is the effect of these measures? Use an ABCDE approach.

This is especially important when the referral is to a specialist service, because the delivery of good care early will help to ensure that the child arrives in the best possible condition. It is an integral part of the role of the specialist service to provide advice to the referring unit throughout the transfer process.

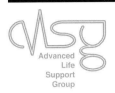

What is needed (from the listener) – again

As the statement of need is so important, it is recommended that it be restated at the end of the communication – allowing the other party to summarise what they perceive is the need is a very useful technique to confirm the success of the communication.

COMMUNICATION METHODS

The communication methods used during the transfer process are the same as those used during day-to-day practice. The usual method within the clinical area instigating the transfer is face-to-face speech, whereas most other communications (within both the referring hospital and the receiving unit) are by telephone. In some areas telemedicine facilities may be available and may aid communication. Occasionally it will be necessary to use radios.

WRITTEN RECORDS

Written records are especially important from both clinical and legal perspectives. Apart from a few taped calls, written notes are usually the only records that remain once the transfer is completed. They must be as accurate as possible and should include as a minimum:
- Child's details
- Timings (date/time of contact, transport and critical events)
- Clinical baseline history and examination
- Clinical interventions and effects of these
- Investigations carried out and their results
- Condition during transfer
- Names of responsible clinicians at each stage of the transfer
- Parent details
- Signature and designation of recording clinician.

(See Chapter 20 and Appendix D for more details about documentation.)

SUMMARY

Clear and effective communication and documentation are an essential part of the transfer process.

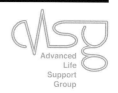

CHAPTER 5

Evaluation

LEARNING OBJECTIVES

In this chapter you will learn about:
- How to recognise and agree to the need for transfer
- How to evaluate the transfer category

Evaluation is a dynamic process that starts from the first contact with the child. The aims are to decide whether transfer is appropriate and, if it is, the urgency with which it needs to be undertaken. By the time that the assessment, control and communication have all been completed, enough information should have been gathered to complete the evaluation.

RECOGNITION OF AND AGREEMENT ON THE NEED FOR TRANSFER

The possibility of transfer on clinical grounds should occur to the team at the referring hospital as the diagnosis unfolds. This requires the recognition that the needs of the child may be better met elsewhere. To make this decision the likely, or possible, diagnosis must be identified and the best treatment for the condition must be known. The lack of local facilities, resources or personnel to make a definitive diagnosis and/or treat the condition optimally must be recognised, and suitable acceptable alternatives need to be available. Referral patterns and common indications for clinical transfers will be well known in most units. Most paediatric transfers will be for ongoing support in a critical care environment (high dependency unit [HDU] or paediatric intensive care unit [PICU]). At the current time there is little provision for specialist transfer of HDU children in the UK as PICU services are not resourced to transfer these children. The situation for neonates is not dissimilar to the paediatric population, although a significant proportion of neonates are also transferred for routine investigation or non-acute treatment, consequently placing a different demand on neonatal transport services.

After identifying the possible need for transfer, the duty clinician at the receiving centre should be contacted. A two-way dialogue will usually result in an agreement that transfer is appropriate. Sometimes immediate agreement is not possible and further information is required. For example, a neurosurgeon may

Paediatric and Neonatal Safe Transfer and Retrieval: The Practical Approach, Edited by Steve Byrne, Steve Fisher, Peter-Marc Fortune, Cassie Lawn and Sue Wieteska. © 2008 Blackwell Publishing, ISBN: 978-1-4051-6919-6.

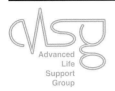

need to assess a computed tomography (CT) scan transmitted electronically from the referring centre. Occasionally agreement is not achieved. This may be because of either hopeless prognosis or the referral being considered inappropriate by the receiving unit. Such decisions must only be taken after discussions between consultants. These deliberations should be meticulously recorded in the notes of both centres as a source for review at a later date.

Usually, after agreement about the appropriateness of transfer, the receiving clinician must check that the centre is physically able to accept the child. In some regions the transport service is independent of any one hospital. They accept the referral and then will locate the nearest suitable bed. Consideration must be given to ensure that the receiving centre is able to deliver the likely required level of care – for example, cardiac surgical support. An exception to this rule might be when the nearest receiving centre has the capability to perform a life-saving surgical intervention that is time critical. In such a situation, transfer before availability of resources may be justified, but the specialist receiving centre will have to arrange further transfer postoperatively.

THE TRANSFER CATEGORY

This is the next stage in the process and represents the outcome of the evaluation. The need for extra treatment before or during transfer should be discussed and an assessment of the urgency of transfer made. The primary goal of safe transfer is to have the appropriate level of care for the child throughout the journey. Thus, for transfer of a child to intensive care, the ambulance should function as a mobile ICU.

It is important to note that, although intensive care children are usually the most complicated (often requiring ventilation and invasive monitoring), they are not necessarily the most time critical. Careful stabilisation before transfer is important.

A useful tool for determining the appropriate transfer needs is the transfer category table shown in Table 5.1. The child's illness or injury is identified in such a way as to incorporate severity and urgency. It provides a consistent method of allocating resources (vehicle, escorts and equipment) and defining the ambulance response time.

The clinical urgency is divided into five categories (Box 5.1). As a rule of thumb the team should be mobilised within 30 minutes for emergency transfers and within 2 hours for urgent transfers.

Box 5.1 Categories of clinical urgency

- Emergency (time critical):
  - unstable
  - stable
- Urgent:
  - unstable
  - stable
- Elective

Emergency – (time critical)

Time critical transfers involve children requiring the most urgent transportation. An example would be a child being involved in a road traffic accident, with

Category of Clinical Incident		Urgency	Vehicle	Driving Speeds	Personnel
Emergency	Unstable	TIME CRITICAL Mobilise team in < 30 minutes local team may need to be mobilised sooner	Transport team ambulance or '999' front line vehicle. Consider air transfer if this significantly reduces journey time without engendering significant delay	Use of blue lights and sirens to maintain normal progress advised. Driving with exceptions may be indicated.	Competent Neonatal/ Paediatric Transport Clinician and Nurse. Occasionally local team to avoid delay
	Stable	TIME CRITICAL Mobilise team in < 30 minutes	Transport team ambulance or '999' front line vehicle. Consider air transfer if this significantly reduces journey time without engendering significant delay	Use of blue lights and sirens to maintain normal progress advised. Driving with exceptions may occasionally be indicated.	Competent Neonatal/ Paediatric Transport Clinician and Nurse. Occasionally local team to avoid delay
Urgent	Unstable	Transfer within 4 hours	Transport team ambulance or '999' front line vehicle if team vehicle not available and significant risk of deterioration	Use of blue lights and sirens to maintain normal progress may be indicated. Normal road speeds	Competent Neonatal/ Paediatric Transport Clinician and Nurse
	Stable	Transfer within 4 hours	Transport team ambulance or other appropriate ambulance e.g. PTS vehicle/'999' ambulance	Normal road speeds	Competent Neonatal/ Paediatric Transport Clinician and Nurse
Elective		Arranged 1-2 days in advance	Transport team ambulance or other appropriate ambulance e.g. PTS vehicle/'999' ambulance	Normal road speeds	Transport Nurse and/or Transport Clinician dependent on clinical situation

Table 5.1 Transfer category table.

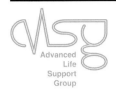

evidence of an expanding intracranial bleed and no resources to operate on site. Children falling into this category are one group for whom consideration should be given to authorising the ambulance driver to exceed speed limits and cross red lights.

Emergency (time critical) – stable

A child in this category will have a secure airway, be cardiovascularly stable and have good venous access. No obvious danger of cardiorespiratory collapse should be present; if it is the child would fall into the unstable group. For these time-critical stable children further delays to refine treatment are likely to offer little or no benefit, and may indeed cause additional harm. If not already booked, an ambulance should be requested either via a 999 call or with an equivalent urgency. In practice it will usually be possible to book transport during the resuscitation/CT scan phase and have it standing by for transfer.

Emergency (time critical) – unstable

Children in this category present the greatest challenge. It may be that with appropriate intervention the unstable child may be stabilised and move into the stable category. However, there will be other occasions where this is not the case. This may be a category where you would consider moving a child who is not comprehensively resuscitated – for example, a newborn with severe persistent pulmonary hypertension. Despite all efforts, including nitric oxide (NO) therapy, the child may remain cardiovascularly unstable and poorly oxygenated. The decision to transfer may have to be taken in a child who is not fully stabilised in order to instigate ECMO (extracorporeal membrane oxygenation) therapy.

Once all efforts to stabilise the child have been exhausted, the team leader, in communication with both referring and receiving consultants, must first consider whether, on balance, it is appropriate to move the child. Whatever the outcome of this decision, it must be shared frankly with the child's family. It must also be made clear that, if the transfer is undertaken, there is a significant risk of death en route. Provided that the parents consent to transfer, appropriate transfer should be arranged as soon as possible. If an air transfer will significantly reduce the journey time without engendering a major delay, it should also be considered. Finally the team should consider offering space in the vehicle to at least one parent when there may be a significant risk of death en route. This requires very careful consideration when the medical needs of a recently delivered mother must also be taken into account.

Urgent – stable

Children in this group have been admitted with an acute problem and stabilised by the local team. Most neonatal transfers fall into this category. Although definitive treatment will have been provided, they require transfer for ongoing critical care that is not available locally. A child who has been successfully intubated and ventilated after admission with upper airway obstruction caused by laryngotracheobronchitis would be a good example of this. Arrangements should be made to move the child within a period of 1–2 hours. Provided that there is no danger of compromising the child's care, both referral and retrieval teams should be flexible on timing in order to optimise the use of each other's staff and the ambulance staff.

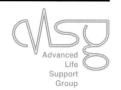

Urgent – unstable

In common with the time-critical–unstable children, this group presents a significant challenge. These children may require HDU rather than ICU care but be at significant risk of deteriorating – for example, a child with a long history of ICU admissions secondary to a poor respiratory reserve, currently in moderate respiratory distress and requiring supplementary oxygen who had received previous management by non-invasive ventilation.

Such children require expert evaluation of their current status. The risks and benefits of intubating the child and moving them into the *urgent–stable* group should be considered. If it is decided that transport should proceed without intubation, it is essential that a person with appropriate airway skills accompanies the child as an escort. A senior clinician may be required, depending on the perceived risk and the expected duration of the journey.

Elective

Many neonatal and a number of paediatric transfers are arranged for elective procedures or investigations. There are no acute physiological considerations that are likely to require significant intervention during transfer – for example, a 6-week-old, preterm (28 weeks) baby, on supplementary oxygen, being transferred for treatment of retinopathy of prematurity. Such transfers should usually be arranged 1 or 2 days in advance. Final confirmation of the availability of a cot/operative facilities, at the receiving centre should be made on the day of transfer. Referring and receiving centres must be crystal clear with regard to the expected stay, requirement for supporting staff and access to piped gas and electricity supply. For example, an ICU at a receiving centre may make a bed space available for the referring NICU team to care for a baby for a few hours while investigations are carried out, with a clear agreement that the baby will return, with the referring hospital team, to their referring centre, once investigations are complete.

SUMMARY

Evaluation of the child is a continuous process that starts from first medical contact. It aims to determine the rationale for and the urgency of transfer.

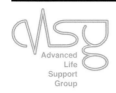

CHAPTER 6

Preparation and packaging

LEARNING OBJECTIVES

In this chapter you will learn about:
- How to prepare the child, equipment and personnel for transfer
- How to package the child for transfer

INTRODUCTION

It is not possible to provide all critical care treatment modalities during a transfer. However, the standards of monitoring and management should not be reduced unless the overall benefits of change outweigh the increase in risk. In fact, with adequate preparation, most advanced care procedures can continue throughout. To achieve this, both the current needs of the child and their potential needs en route must be considered. Before leaving, everything must be packaged, by fully protecting and securing both the child and all equipment. Appropriate measures to minimise the deleterious effects of the hostile environment should also be undertaken.

Preparation and packaging does not only involve the physical preparation and continued treatment of the child, but also the preparation and packaging of the accompanying clinical staff. All the equipment that is required to monitor and treat the child during transportation must be gathered, tested and packed. This is whether the child is to travel on a bed, trolley, transport incubator/pod or stretcher, thought must be given in advance to the practicalities of being able to observe and access them and any equipment. It is important to ensure that the whole package is safe for the child and the accompanying staff (Figure 6.1).

PREPARATION

There are three distinct components to preparation before packaging can be commenced. First, where possible, the child must be stabilised to reduce physiological complications during the journey; second, all the necessary equipment must be found and checked; finally, the personnel who are to undertake the transfer must be fully prepared.

Paediatric and Neonatal Safe Transfer and Retrieval: The Practical Approach, Edited by Steve Byrne, Steve Fisher, Peter-Marc Fortune, Cassie Lawn and Sue Wieteska. © 2008 Blackwell Publishing, ISBN: 978-1-4051-6919-6.

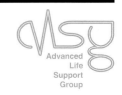

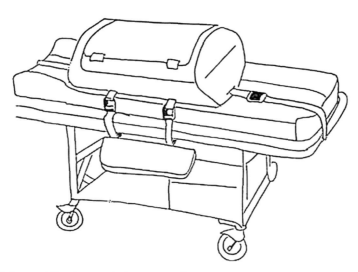

Fig. 6.1 Baby pod fixed to ambulance stretcher.

Child preparation

Before the transfer takes place the team leader must ensure that the child is in the best possible condition and that all team members are fully briefed about his or her needs.

Once again the ABCDE approach is used. The child must have a 'definitive' airway. If there is any doubt about the child's airway or conscious level, elective intubation should be considered and undertaken before departure. A decision to omit intubation in these circumstances must involve the consultant in charge of the retrieval. Most children requiring transfer will be intubated. The need to intubate en route should ideally never arise.

In paediatric trauma the cervical spine must be immobilised in all children unless a full clinical and radiological exclusion of cervical spine injury has been possible (by an appropriate clinician). If in any doubt always immobilise the cervical spine. A size-appropriate hard collar, blocks and tapes or straps should be used. Simple measures such as bags of fluid placed either side of the head or makeshift collars are completely unsuitable for the transfer environment. Children without a history of trauma often need their head stabilised during transfer for both comfort and the security of their airway; a vacuum mattress is ideal for this purpose (Figure 6.2).

Spontaneously breathing children may require a non-re-breathing mask with high-flow oxygen. Conscious children may be better transferred sitting up and accompanied by a parent.

Chest drains must be modified for transfer; underwater seal bottles are cumbersome and can tip; one-way valve drainage bags or Heimlich flutter valves should be substituted.

Usually, for paediatric transfers, at least two reliable peripheral, or one sutured central (including umbilical venous catheter or UVC), intravenous line should be available. For larger children on shorter transfers maintenance fluids may sometimes be omitted. An infusion pump or syringe driver will be far more effective than a drip set at low rates, whilst enroute. Syringe drivers are a less cumbersome alternative usually well suited to neonates and children.

Infusions should be rationalised to reduce their number to a minimum. If necessary many sedatives and muscle relaxants can be given by bolus injection or mixed in one syringe.

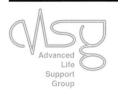

(a)

(b)

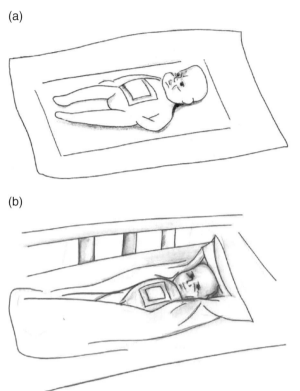

Fig. 6.2 Vacuum mattress: (a) deflated; (b) inflated.

Any suspicion of a spinal injury, at any level, warrants appropriate spinal immobilisation during transport. This makes handling of the child much easier. Spinal boards must be secured to the ambulance stretcher to CEN standards. All fractures should be immobilised before transport to minimise pain, further damage and blood loss. Be aware that some fixators and traction devices may not fit into the transport vehicle and may require modification or removal.

A multidisciplinary, detailed observation chart should be started as early as possible.

Children easily become hypothermic while being resuscitated and stabilised for transfer. Warm air quilts and/or warming mattresses (such as a chemical gel mattress, for example, Transwarmer) should be considered early on, and efforts should be made to minimise the time spent exposed during invasive procedures in order to reduce heat losses. If the child has undergone a cerebral injury the optimal target temperature should be discussed with the receiving centre.

Equipment preparation
Child equipment

Transport equipment should not be used for any other purpose. It should be stored in a specific location and must be checked regularly (preferably at least daily). Monitors and pumps must be kept fully charged. Some items may be stored separately – for example, drugs that are stored cold, warmed fluids, controlled drugs and batteries that are on charge. These can easily be forgotten and it is therefore important to check everything. A loading checklist is helpful in this regard (see Appendix D).

Many hospitals use transport rucksacks that can be unzipped all the way round and laid out flat. These can hold large amounts of equipment and are very portable. In the confines of an ambulance or aircraft, rucksacks with single compartments can be very awkward to open and access. In these instances multi-compartment bags have proved very successful. A number of these bags also contain smaller pouch-bags with specific roles such as 'airway' or 'intravenous access'. When moving critically ill children over long distances, a great deal of equipment may be required. To spread the load, two smaller transport packs are often better than one large one.

After each transfer, the medical and nursing staff must go through the equipment and check the contents against a list (such as the one in Appendix D), replacing any items used. This is made easier if during a transfer, a record of any items used is kept.

The kit must contain all means of manually supporting the airway, and full intubation equipment. It should include a selection of sizes of airways and endotracheal tubes and, for PICU transfers, an emergency cricothyroidotomy set. Effective portable suction must be available at all times. Hand or foot operated units can be very efficient for large volume suction and have the advantage of needing no external power or gas supply. Be wary of transport incubators that use gas-driven suction because these rapidly deplete oxygen supplies. This is dealt with in more detail in Chapter 9.

The team should ascertain the flow rate of oxygen that is required to deliver adequate ventilation to the child through either a breathing circuit or a ventilator. They must also estimate the total journey time and its component parts. The transfer to the ambulance, the ambulance journey and transfer from ambulance at the other end will each contribute to the overall time. With air retrievals there may be multiple transfers between transport vehicles and delays at airports for landing and take-off. A worst-case scenario for each component will provide the total duration of time that should be covered by the oxygen reserves carried by the team.

Ideally, for children requiring ventilatory support, a mechanical ventilator should be used. This must be durable, safe and reliable. Many of the suitable portable ventilators are oxygen driven with a variable gas mix that provides between 21 and 100% oxygen. All ventilators have tables available detailing their gas consumption.

Transport ventilators such as the Babypac, Ventipac and Oxylog consume oxygen at different rates depending on the set ventilatory parameters.

All ICU children require a ventilator that can cope with a variety of pulmonary states. PEEP (positive end-expiratory pressure) is essential for all children's transfers.

The estimated oxygen requirements should be calculated and the figure obtained then doubled to allow for unexpected delays, etc. The number of cylinders required is calculated by dividing estimated consumption by cylinder capacity (see Chapter 9). If this calculation yields one cylinder or less, always take a second one. Ensure that all cylinders already in the ambulance are fully secured and full at the start of the transfer.

Ensure that, in the event of a ventilator failure, it is possible to ventilate a child. This will require either a second cylinder with the appropriate connections or a combination regulator that has provision for Shräder *and* nipple outlets.

For unusually long road transfers, the ambulance may have to stop en route at a hospital or ambulance station to collect more oxygen. A reserve is therefore

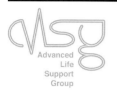

especially important when transporting from isolated locations, where additional supplies cannot be collected during the journey.

Specialised transfers may require further equipment checks, for example incubators, NO or specialised ventilation such as high-frequency jet ventilation (HFJV).

Staff equipment and packaging

All the transport team must be adequately equipped to cope with the weather both from a safety perspective and to ensure that they are comfortable. Tired, hungry and travel-sick staff are not in the best position to provide the high standard of care that the child needs during transfer. Some members of the transfer team may experience motion sickness, which can easily impair their performance during a transfer. Staff who suffer from motion sickness may benefit from a variety of treatments and remedies.

All transport team members must have access to a protective high-visibility jacket. This should be worn when outside the safety of the hospital or the ambulance. The team should have the ability to communicate by mobile telephone (with both the receiving and the home unit) and the resources to ensure that they can make their own way back to the base if necessary.

It is not unknown for satellite navigation systems to fail, so a map is essential, particularly when travelling outside the region. In the event of a long journey, food and refreshment should be carried together with the resources either to get home or to stay overnight in safe accommodation.

Personnel preparation

Staff involved in transport should be trained in the use of all equipment and drugs being used. They should have appropriate life support skills for both the current and possible needs of the child. Good communication between transport staff is essential in order to maximise efficiency and minimise risk.

Packaging the child

The key words in packaging the child are security and accessibility.

Any endotracheal (ET) tube must be securely fastened. In children this usually means fixation with Elastoplast or Sleek, using an accepted method (see Chapter 10). A nasal rather than an oral tube may provide greater stability for transportation and is easier to secure. However, nasal intubation is a skilled procedure and should not be attempted, without good reason, in an unwell child. It is rarely appropriate to reintubate children nasally if they are already stable and ventilated through an appropriately secured oral ET tube. In neonates there are several commercially available tube-fixing systems and usually these are then attached to a well-fitting hat. This also has the advantage of reducing heat loss from the head.

Excessively long tubes may kink, especially when attached to a ventilator circuit. Small-sized paediatric tubes are at much greater risk of this. However, an uncut tube does provide an additional degree of safety if the ventilator tubing is snagged and may be considered. ET tubes should never be cut down until a chest radiograph has confirmed that they are long enough.

When the child is being transferred, the ET tube must be protected, at all times, to prevent extubation. This is a particular risk when moving from bed to stretcher, or incubator to transport incubator. Most children will tolerate a short period of disconnection. This is the safest way to avoid inadvertent extubation during such

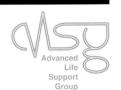

manoeuvres. During paediatric transfers end-tidal carbon dioxide (ETCO$_2$) should be monitored at all times. This provides information on effectiveness of ventilation and is a sensitive disconnection alarm.

If the atmospheric pressure is likely to change significantly, for example, during air transport, the cuff on a cuffed tube should be filled with water rather than air. This avoids the associated volume changes that may damage the trachea.

The eyes of sedated children should be protected by closing the lids with tape or Geliperm. This will prevent accidental corneal abrasion, but must still allow visualisation of the pupils, to assess sedation levels and signs of raised intracranial pressure (ICP).

Ventilators and associated equipment need thorough checking before departure. All members of the transport team must be familiar with the particular ventilator in use. The ventilator should be fastened securely to the side of the stretcher, incubator or pod. It must be clearly visible and easy to reach at all times. The contents gauge of the oxygen supply must also be clearly visible and monitored regularly. A reserve oxygen supply must be readily to hand and should have an appropriate connector attached. A cylinder key is an essential part of the kit and should be readily available. Ventilators and cylinders must be securely fastened for transport.

Adequacy of respiratory support is assessed by pulse oximetry and capnography in all children and some neonates. The oximeter probe can be placed on a finger inside under the blankets because, in this low light, it is more likely to work well. There is little doubt that pulse oximeters using Masimo SET technology vastly reduce the deleterious effects of movement and vibration during transport. Ventilator pressure and disconnect alarms are notoriously difficult to hear during transport. If fitted, they should be used but must not be considered an adequate indicator of problems on their own. Vigilance and ETCO$_2$ monitoring are the most reliable method.

When the child is packaged before transfer, one point of venous access should be kept easily available for administering drugs and fluids. Jugular, subclavian and umbilical central lines often provide good points of access for a carer sitting at the head of the child. The access port can be secured to the shoulder of the child to avoid displacement during the journey, or be just outside the incubator/baby pod for babies.

Many parameters need to be monitored to assess the child's physiological status. This results in a potentially huge jumble of cables and wires. To avoid this all the leads should be brought together as one bundle, which can be protected with cable ties. This is also a problem for babies in a transport incubator and it is well worth taking several minutes to untangle and organise lines and leads before transfer of the baby.

Invasive pressure lines must be flushed and zeroed before use. They are accurate, less sensitive to vibration and rapidly detect changes in pressure. However, they must be kept bubble free and secured at an appropriate level relevant to the child. Sets are now available that do not require cumbersome pressure bags. Ensure that they are readily accessible for flushing and zeroing. After securing the transducers, all the connections in the pressure set should be retightened to avoid disconnection en route.

The power for monitors and pumps can often be drawn from the ambulance. This may require prior discussion with the transport vehicle operator.

There are now commercial systems available (such as the I-Stat system) that will allow near-child testing of blood gases and electrolytes en route if required.

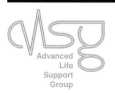

Heat loss presents a major problem, particularly outside the warm hospital environment, and can be substantially reduced by covering children. They can be wrapped in pre-warmed blankets and then covered with an insulating layer. Alternatively, special quilts or sleeping bags can be used for maximal insulation and Transwarmer mattresses can provide an active heat source. These also ensure that, once wrapped, the child is very neatly packaged, avoiding lots of loose leads and lines. However this is achieved, it is vital that it may be quickly removed without risk of snagging lines or the ET tube if access to the child is required in an emergency. The environment inside the transport vehicle should also be considered. It may be possible to heat or cool this.

Fixing of stretchers, incubators or baby pods is often ambulance specific and can vary between regions and ambulance services. All fixing mechanisms should be CEN compliant. It is obviously vital that transport teams be kept aware of significant changes to their local ambulance fleets, unless they have their own customised vehicles.

SUMMARY

Adequate preparation of the child, the equipment and the transport personnel, together with attention to packaging, will ensure that the transportation phase itself has the best chance of being free of adverse events.

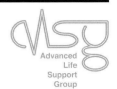
CHAPTER 7

Transportation

INTRODUCTION

Inter-hospital transportation takes place in three distinct phases. First, the child is moved from the referring unit to the transferring vehicle. Second, the vehicle, team and child move from the referring unit to the receiving unit. Finally, the child is moved from the transferring vehicle to the receiving unit incubator, bed or cot. In the first and last phases the child is transferred from bed/incubator to trolley, incubator, pod or vice versa. These transfers represent a period of increased risk of incident unless managed very carefully. The three phases are dealt with separately below.

LEAVING THE REFERRING UNIT

The child and transfer team should be fully prepared and packaging must be complete before any movement is initiated. A final check should be carried out to ensure that no actions are required to optimise the child's physiological status. In addition, a final check should be made to ensure that tubes, drains and lines are as secure as possible. A formal checklist is a very helpful aide memoire and should be considered best practice. Box 7.1 illustrates such a list. The very last action to be taken on departure should be disconnection from the hospital power and gas supplies.

Paediatric and Neonatal Safe Transfer and Retrieval: The Practical Approach, Edited by Steve Byrne, Steve Fisher, Peter-Marc Fortune, Cassie Lawn and Sue Wieteska. © 2008 Blackwell Publishing, ISBN: 978-1-4051-6919-6.

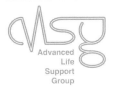

Box 7.1 Checklist before leaving the referring unit

- If breathing spontaneously, change to transport oxygen supply and ensure that mask is appropriate and fitting
- Ensure that the transport oxygen cylinder is full and has the appropriate valve
- If requiring ventilation, attach the child to the transport ventilator to check adequate ventilation and oxygenation are achieved; check blood gases after 10 minutes
- Ensure adequate ventilation on both sides of the chest
- Ensure that any chest drain is secure and functioning
- Ensure that lines are secure, untangled and functioning
- Hang up any fluid bags so that they will not interfere with the transfer of the child
- Check the position of the urinary catheter – make sure that the tube is not kinked
- Check the position of the naso-/orogastric tube
- Plan the move with the team
- Brief the child's parents – give them an opportunity to see and touch their child
- Where appropriate brief the child
- Check that no line or tube is likely to be snared in the move
- Move the child to the transport trolley using appropriate aids

MOVEMENT BETWEEN UNITS

As soon as the child is loaded on to the ambulance, the trolley, incubator or pod should be secured to the vehicle and the security of the child and all equipment checked. The vehicle's gas supplies should be checked and all equipment connected to ambulance gas and power supplies to preserve transport kit resources.

The aim is to provide seamless, appropriate care throughout the transfer. Use a systematic ABCDE approach to identify potential problems that may require action during the transfer. Many potential problems are applicable to any transfer; some are specific to the clinical condition of the individual child. For each of the systems undertake a pre-transfer check before leaving and consider what potential problems may occur. Consideration should be given to how the problems may be avoided and how they can be promptly identified if prevention fails. Where appropriate a plan of action and appropriate equipment should be prepared to deal with each potential scenario.

> **Threats and actions**
> Be prepared, be a pessimist – 'What can go wrong . . . will go wrong!'
> Use an ABCDE approach to:
> - Recognise problems promptly when they arise
> - Ensure that equipment is readily available for anticipated problems
> - Guide pre-planned action

Airway

Before setting off perform a pre-transfer check of the airway (Box 7.2).

Threats to the airway involve a potentially catastrophic total loss of physiological control. The child with an unsecured airway may vomit and aspirate. Endotracheal (ET) tubes may become dislodged, migrate inwards or become blocked with secretions.

> **Box 7.2** Pre-transfer checklist – airway
>
> • Will it be possible to assess the airway during transfer?
> • Is there a member of the team present who can secure that airway, if required?
> • If the child is intubated:
>   – Is the ET tube visible?
>   – Is the length of the tube at the lips/nose recorded?
> • If cuffed, is the pilot balloon visible?
> • Are the connections to the ventilation tubing visible?
> • Is the ventilator tubing secured to ensure that it will not become snared or drag the ET tube out?
> • Does a member of the team have easy access to a prepared pack of the drugs and equipment that might be needed to (re)intubate?

Simple monitoring

Spontaneously breathing children should be covered in such a way that it is possible to continually observe their chest movement and the colour of their face. Listening for sounds of obstructed breathing or ET leaks in a ventilated child is very difficult on the road because of the level of noise within an ambulance. However, despite the problems, basic monitoring techniques should not be abandoned in case of technical failures.

Pulse oximetry and capnography

Pulse oximetry gives a continuous measurement of the level of tissue oxygenation at the probe site. Sometimes, in transfers, the first sign of an airway problem may be a deterioration in the oxygen saturation. However, pulse oximetry can also be adversely affected during transfer. If the child is cold and peripherally vasoconstricted, the signal strength may not be sufficient to give an accurate reading of oxygen saturation. Furthermore, readings can be distorted by vibration artefact and excessive ambient light. The use of Signal Extraction Technology (SET) pulse oximeters, licensed by Masimo, is recommended because they minimise these problems.

Measuring $ETCO_2$ using capnography will give a constant indication of the adequacy of ventilation in the intubated child and should be considered a basic standard in all paediatric transfers. Neonatal teams are also increasingly using this technology because the concerns about excess dead space are not borne out by clinical experience. The capnograph acts as an extremely sensitive disconnection alarm because the trace will disappear as soon as the child is no longer ventilated. This is important as the alarm systems of many transport ventilators leave a lot to be desired. In-line capnographs can be affected by moisture build-up within the sampling window; side-stream capnographs may also cease to work if the sampling tube becomes blocked with moisture. Both pulse oximetry and capnography are described in more detail in Chapter 9.

Threats to the airway

These include the following.

Outward migration of the ET tube – dislodgement

Despite the best efforts to secure it adequately, the ET tube may become dislodged or slip further out. Outward dislodgement of the ET tube will exhibit the signs

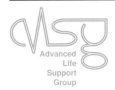

of a leak. An early sign may be a gurgling sound on inspiration, crying or vocalisation; check that the level of the tube at the lips or nose has not changed from the recorded value. As the tube migrates out there may be a loss of the gurgling sound, but also loss of ventilation. Check the ventilation pressure dial and the ETCO$_2$.

ACTION

- Stop the vehicle if possible and assess the child
- Confirm displacement of the tube
- Manually ventilate
- With all the appropriate equipment available, re-position the ET tube or re-intubate and secure the tube

---

Inward migration of the ET tube – endobronchial intubation

Inward migration of the ET tube may show signs similar but not identical to tube obstruction. The first indication may be a drop in pulse oximetry measurements as a result of effectively ventilating only one lung. There may also be an increase in ETCO$_2$ together with subtle changes to the trace. Arrange for the vehicle to slow down and stop as soon as possible. Disconnect from the mechanical ventilator and ventilate by hand. Observe chest movement, listen to breath sounds (if possible) and check the length of the ET tube. If there is clear evidence of migration inwards, withdraw the tube to the correct length. This may be confirmed by direct visualisation. Suction the tube; if there is any difficulty passing a suction catheter it may be blocked (see below). Finally if the tube is patent and correctly placed, consider the possibility of a pneumothorax.

ACTION

- Stop the moving vehicle if possible and assess the child
- Exclude evidence of tube blockage
- Confirm displacement by clinical signs ± direct visualisation
- With all the appropriate equipment available, re-position the ET tube and secure it

---

Endotracheal tube obstruction/occlusion

ET tube 'blockage' as a result of inward migration is discussed above. Small-diameter ET tubes, despite being well secured, can kink, especially when the ventilator tubing is not carefully placed and secured. Obstruction can also occur as a result of secretions within the ET tube. Dry secretions can be a particular problem and arise especially when dry gases are used to ventilate the child. This may be indicated by a decrease in chest movement and/or a prolonged expiratory phase. An urgent attempt should be made to suction the ET tube. Failure to overcome this obstruction can result in inadequate oxygenation and ventilation. The use of a heat moisture exchanger (HME) may reduce this complication.

ACTION

- Stop the moving vehicle if possible and assess the child
- Visually check the ET tube for kinks
- Use the suction device and an appropriate suction catheter to clear secretions from the ET tube lumen
- Consider replacing the ET tube completely

Endotracheal tube cuff leak

Most children are intubated with uncuffed tubes. However, some will have cuffed tubes (Figure 7.1a). The leaking of an inflated cuff of an ET tube can be detected by listening for a gurgling sound on inspiration. This sign will alert the team to the problem. Undetected, a significant loss of inspired minute ventilation will result in hypoventilation, and eventual hypoxia and hypercapnia, as detected by the pulse oximeter and capnograph. A leak around a deflated cuff allows secretions, blood and gastric contents to contaminate the bronchial tree. This may sometimes occur as a result of damage to the pilot balloon. This may be repaired with a cannula threaded into the pilot tube as shown in Figure 7.1b.

(a)

(b)

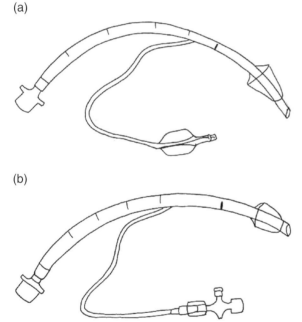

Figure 7.1 Cuffed ET tube: (a) Normal pilot tube; (b) Pilot tube with cannulae inserted proximal to leak.

ACTION

- Stop the moving vehicle if possible and assess the child
- Check that the level of the tube at the lips has not changed from the recorded value
- Attempt to introduce more air/saline into the cuff
- If the pilot balloon is damaged, introduce more air/saline into the cuff and clamp the pilot tube with artery forceps
- If the pilot balloon is lost, consider introducing a 22 G (blue) cannula into the pilot tube and re-inflating the balloon
- Consider replacing the ET tube completely

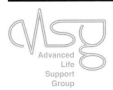

Breathing

Before setting off perform a pre-transfer check of the ventilator (Box 7.3).

As outlined in the airway section, simple monitoring by looking and listening may be difficult to undertake in a moving vehicle. Most transport ventilators display airway pressure on an aneroid dial or digital display. Not all transport ventilators have low- and high-pressure alarms, although these should now be regarded as mandatory. A low-pressure alarm is helpful in suggesting an airway disconnection or leak. High-pressure alarms, when used with pressure-limited, time-cycled ventilators, are unlikely to identify problems in advance of physiological signs.

Box 7.3 Pre-transfer checklist – breathing

Is sufficient oxygen available for the transfer?

Is a self-inflating bag–valve–mask system readily available if required?

If the child is ventilated:

- Is the child settled on, and compliant, with the ventilator?
- Do you have visual, and hands-on access to the ventilator and the breathing circuit?
- Is there symmetrical chest movement?
- Can you see the pulse oximeter and capnograph displays?

Threats to breathing

Pneumothorax

The potential for developing a pneumothorax is higher in certain children. The history can give clues, which should make the team more vigilant. Children with asthma or severe chronic lung disease are at increased risk of developing a pneumothorax. Immunocompromised children with pneumocystis chest infections also fall into this group. Any type of traumatic physical injury as a result of an accident or medical intervention such as thoracic surgery or the placement of a percutaneous internal jugular or subclavian central line will also increase the risk of pneumothorax occurring.

It is important to note that the presence of a pre-existing chest drain can give a false sense of security, because a pleural leak can occur at another site, or the existing chest drain can obstruct. A chest radiograph following central venous pressure line insertion does not exclude the possibility of a pneumothorax developing during transfer. The use of high-inspiratory ventilator pressures will increase the risk of a pneumothorax. Adequate sedation can ensure ventilator compliance and minimise coughing. Both of these may significantly increase intrathoracic pressures, with the concomitant risk of developing an air leak. The use of muscle relaxants during the transfer of an intubated child to minimise the risks of asynchronous respiratory effort and excessive coughing should be considered.

Pneumothorax can be life threatening in a ventilated child but is difficult to confirm in a moving ambulance or aircraft. Noise levels make any attempt to assess air entry into the lung by auscultation extremely difficult. Tracheal shift is an unreliable and very late sign. Hypoxia may be demonstrated by the pulse oximeter together with asymmetrical chest movement. Where measured, a drop in tidal volumes may be observed that may also be associated with a fall in arterial blood pressure secondary to restricted venous return. Where monitored an

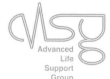

elevated CVP may be seen, which may be associated with a catastrophic fall in blood pressure if a tension pneumothorax develops. If you suspect that a pneumothorax is developing, stop the ambulance, and look and percuss for hyperresonance (Box 7.4). In small children transillumination of the chest might be useful in diagnosis. The treatment of a pneumothorax is discussed in some detail in Chapter 11.

Box 7.4 Pneumothorax detection in the transfer of a ventilated child

- Have a high index of suspicion in children with risk factors
- Investigate promptly any changes in oxygenation or blood pressure
- Exclude a blocked or kinked ET tube
- Check any existing chest drain is not kinked
- Stop the ambulance and undertake a thorough check for hyperresonance and increased transillumination

---

As an emergency measure, a large cannula connected to a 10 ml syringe may be inserted into the second intercostal space in the midclavicular line on the suspected side, or the side demonstrating most hyperresonance. The aim is to perform an emergency decompression of the chest. If a pneumothorax were not present before insertion it would be highly likely to be present afterwards! It is vital that a formal chest drain be inserted as soon as possible. The decompressing cannula should not be removed until a formal chest drain has been inserted. Siting a conventional chest drain during an ambulance journey is fraught with problems; in such circumstances consideration should be given to diverting to a nearby hospital to facilitate the placement. If this is not an option, the use of a chest drain placed with a Seldinger technique may be preferable to a blunt cutdown method.

ACTION

- Stop the ambulance
- Insert a cannula into the second intercostal space in the midclavicular line
- Re-check ventilator and monitors
- Consider diversion to nearby hospital
- Pass a definitive chest drain

Lung ventilation and perfusion mismatch
This occurs during transfer because the blood flow in the relatively low pressure system of the lung is influenced by centripetal and acceleration/deceleration forces. This may result in the child becoming hypoxic. Extra oxygen may need to be added to compensate for increasing intrapulmonary shunting of deoxygenated blood. In the post-premature population this is best managed by a marginal increase in oxygen concentration during transfer. In the premature neonatal population at risk from hyperoxic injury, the oxygen concentration may need to be regularly manipulated to ensure ideal conditions. In either case awareness and vigilance are the keys to mitigating the potential detrimental effects of dynamic mismatching.

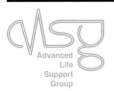

Loss of oxygen supply

Loss of the oxygen supply may not only reduce the oxygen inspiratory concentration (FiO_2) but also stop the transport ventilator working altogether, as many transport ventilators are gas powered. Prevention is much better than cure. Always ensure that you have sufficient supplies to cover the worst-case scenarios for journey time, plus a contingency for unexpected events (see Chapter 9).

Box 7.5 Prevention of loss of oxygen supply

- Calculate the amount of oxygen for each part of the journey before departing
- Check that the required supplies are available
- Know where the cylinder key is stored
- Have a self-inflating bag available at all times

Circulation and organ perfusion

Powerful inertial forces are well known to affect the cardiovascular system in healthy individuals. Hypovolaemic children may adversely respond to the small inertial forces experienced transiently during ambulance transfer, as a result of rapid venous pooling of blood in the peripheral tissues. Although there is little research, it is known that volume loading of the potentially hypovolaemic child reduces the incidence of tachycardia and reduced cardiac output. Hypovolaemia in neonates is fairly rare. Always ensure, where possible, that the child is adequately fluid resuscitated before transfer. The team should bear in mind that overaggressive fluid resuscitation, in the face of active bleeding, may actually increase blood loss, so, during resuscitation, the transfer team will have to balance the concepts of permissive hypotensive resuscitation against the adverse effects of inertia on the hypovolaemic child. This judgement will require expert senior guidance.

It is important for the transfer team to have access to a range of monitoring parameters in order to evaluate the effects of the transfer environment on organ perfusion and the cardiovascular system (Box 7.6).

Box 7.6 Pre-transfer checklist – circulation

- Can you assess the child's circulatory situation?
- Do you have adequate intravenous access?
- Can you respond to changes in the child's circulatory status (inotropes/volume)?

The ECG should be monitored routinely during critical care transfer. At least three electrodes are required, allowing two for sensing and one for grounding. To minimise artefacts these leads should be placed on the thorax and abdomen, not the limbs. They should also be accessible because they commonly become displaced during transfer. Some monitors use more electrodes to allow flexible switching between leads.

Invasive arterial blood pressure is preferable for the transfer of all but the most stable intensive care unit (ICU) transfers. Non-invasive blood pressure cuff readings do not give a 'real-time' view of changes in blood pressure. Each reading is just a snapshot in time and the child's status between readings may change significantly. Cuff pressure readings are often unreliable and distorted by excessive vibration. The air pump in the system also represents a significant drain on the

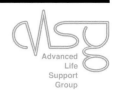

monitor's power source and therefore its battery life. It is more effective to monitor cardiovascular parameters by using invasive pressure lines. Direct arterial pressure monitoring gives the transfer team immediate information. In many children, monitoring invasive CVPs will provide additional useful information on the road. Transducers should be secured to the child at an appropriate level because access may be impossible during the transfer (see Chapter 9).

CVP is measured using the same technology as invasive arterial pressure. If the transport monitor has two invasive pressure channels, both may be displayed en route. If only one is available, arterial monitoring is generally more valuable. Even in this situation, the CVP may be measured intermittently by switching momentarily from the arterial trace, using a male-to-male connector to connect the three-way taps on the arterial and venous tubing.

Urine output measurements should be continued during transfer. When catheterised the hourly urine output should be monitored throughout the transfer as a measure of organ (renal) perfusion.

Core temperature monitoring (for example, nasopharyngeal, oesophageal, axillary or rectal) should be undertaken in all critical care transfers and considered during transfer.

Cardiovascular threats

These include cardiac rhythm disturbances, sudden changes in blood pressure and loss of monitoring. It is outside the scope of this book to give a detailed description of the causes and treatment of all the cardiovascular problems that can occur during transfer. However, Table 7.1 demonstrates a logical structure for identifying a few of these potential cardiovascular problems.

Table 7.1 Structure for identifying some potential cardiovascular problems

	Sign	Threat
Heart rate	Tachycardia	Hypovolaemia pain/awareness
	Bradycardia	Hypoxia raised intracranial pressure
Rhythm	Dysrhythmias	Electrolyte disturbance
		Hypovolaemia (supraventricular/sinus tachycardia)
Blood pressure	Hypotension	Hypovolaemia
		Fault in inotrope delivery
	Hypertension	Pain/awareness

Loss of invasive monitor waveforms
Any invasive line can obstruct with thrombus if not flushed effectively. If a pressure waveform disappears from the screen, the child should be checked for other signs of clinical deterioration immediately before investigating the monitor.

ACTION

- Check that syringe pumps are delivering appropriate volumes of flush or pressure bags are inflated to an appropriate level
- Make sure that all the connections along the flush line are secure to the transducer
- Check that the transducer will register a pressure rise when the line is flushed manually
- Ensure that the cable interface to your monitor is connected

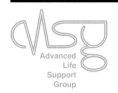

Monitor or syringe pump power failure

All monitors and pumps can potentially suffer power failure in transit. Some pumps allow the replacement of batteries with spares. It is vital to recognise that older NiCd batteries will fail to hold charge to the full extent of the quoted duration. When planning the transfer, consider using a 12 V DC to 240 V AC inverter to allow access to the ambulance battery on transfers.

ACTION

- Replace batteries if practicable
- Sacrifice a less essential infusion drug and swap syringe drivers
- Use any monitoring resources available in the ambulance
- Resort to basic 'look, listen and feel' monitoring

Disability

Rapid changes in acceleration and deceleration forces may result in rises in intracranial pressure (ICP) that can compromise cerebral perfusion. Maintaining a constant speed and minimising sudden turns or harsh braking are therefore beneficial when transferring a child with a traumatic brain injury. Even if the child's cervical spine has been cleared radiologically, it is good practice to secure the child in head blocks to avoid twisting or turning of the head and neck, which may impair venous drainage from an already compromised brain. Limb fractures should be splinted because this may help to reduce pain. Ensure that analgesia is not overlooked in the desire to reduce the number of syringe pumps; local anaesthetic blockade should be considered in the case of rib or limb fracture.

Appropriate sedation must be maintained at all times. Awareness during transfer is very frightening for an incapacitated child in the company of strangers. Despite detailed assessment and resuscitation, occasionally children may undergo a rapid deterioration and even die during the transfer. The team should be aware of this possibility and plan accordingly. Where there is a significant possibility of death very serious consideration should be given to transporting one of the child's parents with the team, even if this is not the standard practice of your centre.

The apparently sedated or unconscious child needs continuing neurological assessment during the transfer. It is embarrassing, to say the least, when staff at the receiving hospital identify a major pupillary change that has not been noted by the transferring team. The position of the eyes and response of the pupils may be the only clinical sign available to confirm elevated ICP. In addition, the only evidence of an underlying convulsion in the paralysed child may be abnormally responding pupils. A member of the transfer team should be positioned so as to be able to inspect pupillary responses to light. A bright handheld light source should be available for this.

If the ICP is being monitored beforehand, it may be possible to continue this during transfer. Intraparenchymal devices, inserted directly into superficial brain tissue through a small hole drilled in the skull, are commonly used to measure ICP. The ICP monitoring system may have an adequate battery for transfer. Many neurosurgical centres use different devices, so compatibility of equipment after transfer may be an issue affecting whether or not to insert such a monitor immediately before transfer. Checking pupil responses, although clearly less discriminating than ICP, should still be regarded as part of the neurological monitoring during transfer even if an ICP monitor is in use. Ideally, the degree of paralysis as a result of muscle relaxant therapy should be monitored with a nerve stimulator. However, access to limbs may be limited and facial twitches can be difficult to interpret during transit. A detailed description of the monitoring of ICP and neuromuscular blockade is outside the scope of this book.

Disability threats

Within the disability part of the assessment structure, threats include a failure of the delivery of sedation, analgesia or muscle relaxant drugs (Box 7.7).

Box 7.7 Pre-transfer checklist – disability

- Does the child require analgesia?
- Assess the child's neurological status in the ambulance
- Plan how the team will respond to changes in the child's neurological status

---

Sweating, tachycardia, hypertension and coughing may all be signs that the level of sedation or analgesia is not adequate. It is important to rule out critical problems with the cardiovascular system. To ensure that an ET tube can be tolerated, the child must be adequately sedated (and paralysed when necessary). Coughing and non-compliance with the ventilator in the presence of a patent ET tube indicate the need to check that sedative and analgesic medications are being delivered.

ACTION

- Check the integrity and patency of associated intravenous lines
- Check correct functioning of any syringe drivers delivering sedation and analgesia
- Replace batteries if practicable
- Sacrifice a less essential infusion drug and swap syringe drivers

---

Exposure and environment

The transporting vehicle can be a hostile place for both child and transfer personnel. Low ambient temperature may result in hypothermia because a thermo-neutral environment is often difficult to achieve. Neonates may be afforded some protection by transport in an incubator or pod. The number of times that such devices are opened should be kept to a minimum, especially in cold weather. Children's temperatures can fall further during the process of moving to and from vehicles and these periods should be carefully managed to minimise exposure to adverse temperature (Box 7.8).

Box 7.8 Pre-transfer checklist – exposure and environment

- Has the child been kept warm during assessment and stabilisation?
- Is the child adequately covered and secured (on stretcher or in pod/incubator)?
- Is the monitoring and therapeutic equipment adequately secured?
- Are all personnel going to be adequately secured?

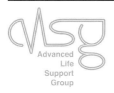

There is a constant threat from unsecured equipment during transfer. It is therefore essential that all equipment be stowed away when not in use. Any equipment and supply boxes must be strapped securely to the stretcher or surrounding framework of the ambulance. All personnel must wear seat belts at all times, unless the vehicle has come to a complete stop. If planning has achieved its aim, the team should have easy, visible and tactile access to all important component parts of the child and monitoring package. Any emergency procedure that will require a team member to leave his or her seat should be undertaken only when the ambulance is at a standstill.

ACTION

- Is emergency clinical intervention required?
- Can action be undertaken from the seat while secured?
- If not, prepare to stop the ambulance to deal with the emergency

---

ARRIVING AT THE RECEIVING UNIT

The arrival and handover procedure should follow the ACCEPT structure, although the order of some of the components may be changed and the concept of evaluation reverts to the normal understanding of the word and its association with reflective practice (Table 7.2).

Table 7.2 Use of ACCEPT in handover

ACCEPT	Use of ACCEPT in handover
Assessment	Combine assessment and 'a summary of the transfer process'
Control	The handing over of control
Communication	Communicate the 'history of the transfer and the evaluation'
Evaluation	Reflect on the whole of the transfer process
Preparation and packaging	Unpack the child
Transportation	Transfer the child

Before arriving at the receiving unit repeat the steps undertaken in assessment (page 17). Remember the 'sound bite' and the systematic approach to the problems and the actions taken. The team should be in a position to reflect on the transfer and to make a general evaluation of the process so far. This assessment and evaluation combined will enable the team to communicate what is a complex story in a concise and clear fashion.

While the transferring team leader is still in control, there is a need to agree when the receiving unit's team leader will take over. This should occur only after a full handover has taken place, following which the child has been safely transferred on to the receiving unit's bed and attached to the ventilator. Only then should the receiving team take full responsibility for the child's care. There is then a 'grey area', during which monitoring and syringe-driver medications are transferred to the receiving unit's equipment.

'Prepare and package' now becomes 'prepare to unpackage'. A systematic plan for attaching the child to the receiving unit's equipment is agreed as above.

Unpacking, and executing the actual transfer of the child, requires team work. The whole procedure needs to be risk assessed, and a plan formulated and executed under the control of one or other team leader. Special care needs to be taken during this transfer to ensure that tubes, drains and lines are not dislodged during the transfer from the trolley or incubator to the ICU bed, incubator or cot. One example of assessing risk is shown in Box 7.9.

Box 7.9 Example of risk assessment

The assessment shows there is a significant risk of ET tube dislodgement during the transfer from stretcher to bed.
The plan might be:
- Check that the ET tube is still secure
- Check that the level of the tube at the lips has not changed from the recorded value
- Allocate a team member to hold the ET tube
- Consider disconnecting the child from the breathing circuit for the period of the move
- Consider not disconnecting but ensure that breathing circuit is not going to drag on the ET tube

Implementation: if the team leader agrees then the plan is executed

---

Before returning to the base hospital, the transfer team should ensure that they have handed over all the case notes, radiographs and laboratory investigations. Many hospitals now collect data on inter-hospital transfers; these forms should be completed and returned to the appropriate place.

Checks should ensure that all medical equipment is returned. Any equipment thought to be faulty should be quarantined and a clear history of the circumstances around the problem should be given to the electrical or biomedical engineers. Any partially used sedation syringes or other unused drugs must be securely disposed of before returning to the ambulance.

SUMMARY

Attention to detail at all three stages of the transfer will ensure that the child is delivered in the best possible condition.

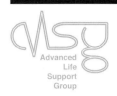

CHAPTER 8

Putting ACCEPT into practice

LEARNING OBJECTIVES

In this chapter you will learn about how the information in Chapters 1–7 can be used to develop a structured approach to transferring children and infants

The preceding chapters have considered each stage of the ACCEPT process in detail. In this chapter, we will work through a practical example of how to pull the aspects of ACCEPT into a cohesive, logical sequence. There is a considerable overlap between ACC and E. These are often processes that will occur simultaneously. However, it is still important mentally to keep them distinct to enable clarity and thoroughness. There will be differences in the way that the ACCEPT principle is applied, depending on whether one is a referrer or a receiver (transport team or unit), although, the overall model remains the same.

The Assessment, Control, Communication and Evaluation steps remain identical whether you are a referrer or receiver.

Communication becomes increasingly complex with increasing numbers of individuals involved. Telephone or video conferencing can be very useful in these circumstances.

When the transfer team is not the referrer an additional handover will need to be undertaken on arrival to the referring centre, which must include:
A: Reassessment, 'What's been done and what needs to be done?'
C: Control – delegating tasks to be done.
C: Communication with professionals and parents; documentation.
E: Further evaluation whether transfer is still appropriate.
Both referrer and receiver will be involved with the preparation, packaging and pre-departure checks, transportation (PPT). Handover at the receiving centre should occur according to the ACCEPT principles.

EXAMPLE

Male infant Robertson is referred from St Elsewhere. He is a term baby and has been cyanosed from birth. He was a normal delivery and was born without any foetal distress. He is currently being managed in a level II neonatal unit at a hos-

Paediatric and Neonatal Safe Transfer and Retrieval: The Practical Approach, Edited by Steve Byrne, Steve Fisher, Peter-Marc Fortune, Cassie Lawn and Sue Wieteska. © 2008 Blackwell Publishing, ISBN: 978-1-4051-6919-6.

pital 20 miles from the local transport team base. A local echocardiogram has shown that he has transposition of the great arteries. He needs to be transferred to the paediatric cardiology centre which is 50 miles north of St Elsewhere. We will examine the transfer process from the perspective of a third party transport team.

Assessment
The problem
A more detailed history establishes that baby Robertson is the third child of a 25-year-old woman who suffers from moderately severe asthma. His older brother has behavioural problems. Baby Robertson is breathing in air with oxygen saturations of 84%. He has no respiratory distress. His heart rate is 130 beats/min and his pH and pCO_2 are within normal ranges. He is 6 hours old and the referring centre has already started a prostaglandin E_2 infusion through a peripheral per-cutaneous long line at 10 ng/kg/min. He has been stable on this for 2 hours. His chest radiograph is unremarkable. The local working diagnosis is transposition of the great vessels.

The sound bite
The relevant information may be summarised quickly as shown in the box.

A 6-year-old stable term male infant, breathing air with oxygen saturations of 84% on a prostaglandin E_2 infusion at 10 ng/kg/min with suspected transposition of the great arteries who needs transfer to a paediatric cardiac surgical centre.

What's being done?
This statement summarises what has actually been done for the child. It should also prompt a structured approach (ABCDE) to what should be done.

The philosophy of primary and secondary survey and immediate resuscitation applies.

Airway: patent and stable

Breathing: satisfactory

Circulation: capillary refill time <2 seconds, heart rate (HR) 130, mean blood pressure (BP) is 45 mmHg. Preductal saturations are 84% in room air

Disability: glucose 6.4 mmol/l

Baby is unsettled and is alert and active. He is not on antibiotics.

Primary survey has been undertaken and no immediate resuscitation is required. A further arterial blood gas analysis, temperature and blood sugar assessment may be needed.

What is needed next is transfer to a paediatric cardiac surgical centre by a suitable team. It is possible that he may need ventilation because of the prostaglandin E_2 infusion and the associated risk of apnoea.

Control
During the assessment stage, the following staff are likely to be involved: children's transport nurse and transport clinician.

The local team are likely to comprise a paediatrician (either consultant or middle grade) and nurses on the local neonatal unit. The team leader is likely to be chosen from the transport team. This person should allocate tasks.

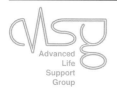

Tasks

The baby is stable, so the next clinical question is to consider the need for intubation. With a low rate of prostaglandin E_2 infusion the risk of apnoea is low; if the infant has been stable on the rate of infusion for 2 hours it is reasonable to transport the infant unventilated. This will need further assessment on arrival of the team. The ability to safely ventilate this infant on the transfer is essential.

The transport team need to review the prostaglandin infusion because such infusions are commonly miscalculated as a result of lack of familiarity with an infrequently used medication and concentration. There is also often confusion over different prostaglandin preparations and the wrong one may be in use.

Equipment should be assembled, including spare medications and an appropriate transport system with ventilator.

Communication

At this stage, all key individuals should be fully informed about the management of the child. In this instance, the following people may be considered appropriate:
- Transport team members including lead clinician
- Referring and receiving unit clinicians; consultant in charge of care
- Paediatric Cardiologist.

It is important to use a structured format for communication:
- Who you are
- What is needed (from the listener)
- What the (relevant) child's details are
- What the problem is
- What has been done to address the problem
- What happened
- What needs to be done next.

A conversation between the transfer clinician (TC) and the receiving unit sister in the PICU may be as shown in the box.

PICU: Hello, Sister Smith here – how can I help?

TC: Hello Sister, my name is Dr Howell. I am on the neonatal transfer team from St Peter's, I would like to transfer a newborn boy from St Elsewhere with suspected transposition of the great arteries to you for further assessment.

PICU: What is the baby's name?

TC: Baby Robertson – he was born at term and is now 6 hours old. He is stable breathing room air with oxygen saturations of 84%. He is on a prostaglandin E_2 infusion at 10 ng/kg per min. He has had an Echo by the local team.

PICU: We do have a bed available at the moment. Can you tell me a bit more about him?

TC: Yes, certainly. His delivery was unremarkable and he didn't need resuscitation at birth. He weighs 3.8 kg. He was noted to be cyanosed shortly after delivery. As I said he is breathing, his saturations are 84% and he is on a prostaglandin E_2 infusion at 10 ng/kg per min via a long line. He has intravenous 10% dextrose running at 60 ml/kg per day and he otherwise appears well. His blood gases are fine

PICU: Is he going to be coming over ventilated?

Continued

TC: No, he is stable at the moment and he has been on prostaglandin for a couple of hours now. We will reassess him when we get there but hopefully we can bring him over extubated – if we are at all concerned we will intubate him. If we do I will ring to let you know.

PICU: Well that all sounds OK. What time do you think you might get to us?

TC: We are going out to St Elsewhere which is 20 miles from here and bringing him up to you. We will probably be with you in about 3–4 hours time. Would that be allright?

PICU: Yes that's fine. I will let the cardiologist and the PICU doctors know – you can contact me on the direct line 020 7555 5555. Please ring us before you leave St Elsewhere.

TC: No problem, I will get back to the referring centre and let them know what we have agreed - I can be contacted via switch 020 8444 4444 on bleep 3134. I will make sure the parents know what is planned.

Obviously a great deal more information could be shared here, but the essential information has been exchanged, the bed negotiated, contact details exchanged and agreement made about who will communicate with whom.

Evaluation

The clinical need for transfer is not in doubt because the infant needs a paediatric cardiology assessment. It is appropriate that he be transferred by the neonatal team.

Category: urgent–stable

Mode: mode of transport needs to be considered – ambulance is appropriate here as transfer times are likely to be acceptable.

Preparation and packaging

Preparation

Preparation should follow the ABCDE format:

- **Airway and Breathing**: there are no concerns about this baby's airway and breathing at present but he is at risk of apnoea, he needs to be assessed carefully when the team arrive. If there is any doubt or his infusion rate of prostaglandin needs to be increased then intubation must be reconsidered.
- **Circulation**: he does not require fluid resuscitation or other cardiovascular support at present. Prostaglandin should be treated like oxygen or inotropes and carried in excess on this transport.
- **Disability and Environment**: although this is a term infant with a good birthweight, he is still very susceptible to cold stress and should therefore be transported in a transport incubator or baby pod. Other elements to preparation include the medical and nursing staff, who need to be informed of all the clinical details. The team must be adequately dressed and prepared (for example, take money).

Prostaglandin E_2 is a critical infusion and should not be stopped at any point during the transfer. Sufficient pumps must be carried to enable all critical infusions and sedation and maintenance to be delivered simultaneously. At least four pumps are likely to be needed for this journey. It is vital to have a multiparameter monitor for this child, ideally comprising heart rate, temperature, pulse oximetry,

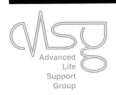

non-invasive and/or invasive blood pressure monitoring (if an arterial line has been placed) and ETCO$_2$.

Packaging

The baby will need to be in a transport incubator or baby pod on a trolley that can be firmly secured to the ambulance. All equipment needs to be firmly fixed and stowed according to CEN regulations. The expected oxygen requirement should be calculated based on the expected duration of the transfer and then doubled. All equipment should be secured to the trolley and all drips and lines must be secured to the baby. It is important not to forget the notes and radio-graphs, and cardiac echo images if possible.

Transfer

Before setting off on a transfer the team leader should consider what could go wrong during this transfer.

They should think about how to observe the child and the electronic monitoring that will be required during transport. Transfer speed should be considered. This is an urgent transfer and the child needs to be cared for in the paediatric cardiology centre, but it is not time critical and the child is currently stable. Therefore normal road speed limits should be observed.

Handover should be a joint exercise between nursing and medical staff and should follow the structured ACCEPT approach. All notes, radiographs and investigations should be handed over before returning transport equipment to the transfer centre for cleaning.

SUMMARY

This example has shown how ACCEPT can be used to facilitate a safe transfer.

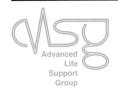

PART III

Practical aspects of paediatric and neonatal transfer medicine

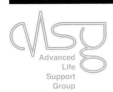

CHAPTER 9

Oxygen therapy and monitoring

LEARNING OBJECTIVES

In this chapter you will learn about:
- The appropriate delivery of oxygen
- The appropriate use of monitors
- The essentials of batteries and power supplies

APPLYING OXYGEN

Oxygen supplies

Cylinders

It is important to have a basic understanding of oxygen supplies. Most oxygen cylinders are made of steel; however, there is a trend away from this traditional material towards 'hood-wrapped' advanced steel carbon fibre (Aramid), better known by trade names such as Kevlar. This is also used in ballistic protective applications such as bullet-proof vests and aircraft body parts.

Lightweight carbon-fibre cylinders are filled to a higher pressure. Steel cylinders are graded by size, the most common ones used in NHS wards and departments being D, E and F sizes (Table 9.1). All UK steel oxygen cylinders are filled to a pressure of 137 bar (1 bar = 1 atm = 14.7 lb/in^2 [p.s.i.] = 101.33 kPa).

For a given temperature there is a linear relationship between the pressure (P) in the cylinder and the volume (V) of the gas (Boyle's law: $P_1 \times V_1 = P_2 \times V_2$). Therefore, as the contents of the cylinder reduce so does the pressure on the gauge. A full E-sized cylinder will contain 680 litres of gas; when the gauge reads half-full, the cylinder will contain 340 l.

If an oxygen flowmeter is set to deliver 10 l/min, a full E-sized cylinder will be empty in 68 min (680/10), and a half-filled E-sized cylinder will be empty in 34 min, after which time there will be no gas or pressure left in the cylinder.

Connections and keys

It is important to understand the component parts of the connections between a gas cylinder and the oxygen delivery system. The pressure in compressed gas cylinders must be reduced before it reaches a flowmeter or ventilator, and this reduction in pressure is accomplished using a regulator. The connection to the regulator may be either a pin-index system or a bull-nosed fitting (Figures 9.1 and 9.2; see Table 9.1).

Paediatric and Neonatal Safe Transfer and Retrieval: The Practical Approach, Edited by Steve Byrne, Steve Fisher, Peter-Marc Fortune, Cassie Lawn and Sue Wieteska. © 2008 Blackwell Publishing, ISBN: 978-1-4051-6919-6.

Table 9.1 Oxygen cylinder characteristics

	D	E	F
Common usage	Portable	Anaesthetic 'machines'	Emergency department trolleys Theatre trolleys
Capacity (l)	340	680	1360
Connection	Pin index	Pin index	Bull nosed

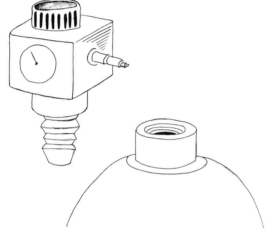

Fig. 9.1 Bull-nosed fittings.

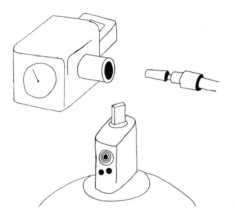

Fig. 9.2 Pin-index fittings.

In the UK all D- and E-sized oxygen cylinders have a pin-index fitting system, which is specific to the medical gas to be supplied. Larger cylinders, F size and above, do not have this gas-specific anti-confusion device. Cylinders containing other medical gases, such as medical air, could be inadvertently connected to the regulator that is meant to supply oxygen.

Oxygen regulators have an output connector either to a flowmeter/nipple for direct connection to green oxygen mask tubing, or to a Schräder connector, which connects to a white pressure hose leading to a ventilator. Similar to the pin-index fitting, the Schräder connector is specific to the medical gas. Newer lightweight cylinders have a built-in combination regulator flowmeter with Schräder and nipple outlets.

Oxygen masks and resuscitation circuits, as described below, must be connected to a regulator and flowmeter with an oxygen nipple outlet. Transport ventilators

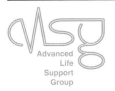

are connected to a regulator via the Schräder outlet. In the event of a ventilator failure, you will either need a second cylinder with the appropriate connections or use a combination regulator that has provision for Schräder and nipple outlets to ensure that you can attach and use a breathing circuit. An example is the STAR valve the BOC lightweight combination regulator shown below (Figure 9.3).

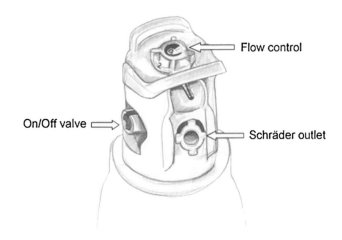

Fig. 9.3 STAR valve.

To plan the requirement for oxygen supplies during a journey, a working knowledge of oxygen masks, breathing circuits and ventilators is necessary.

Oxygen masks are part of everyday life in UK hospitals; they are very much taken for granted, although the theory of operation is often poorly understood by those who use them. The amount of oxygen delivered may vary with the child's respiratory effort.

Variable performance oxygen devices

One of the most common oxygen masks to be seen in hospitals is the Hudson type (Figure 9.4). This clear plastic mask with an oxygen nipple and side holes is designed to deliver up to 50% oxygen in most children. The normal inspiratory flow pattern is approximately sinusoidal; the inspiratory:expiratory time ratio varies from 1:1 to 1:2, and the peak inspiratory flow rate is approximately three to four times the minute volume. The peak inspiratory flow rate is related to the tidal volume.

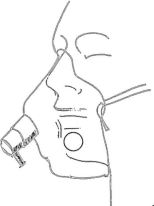

Fig. 9.4 Oxygen mask: Hudson type.

During the first second of inspiration, the child initially breathes in the oxygen mixture from inside the mask. Then air is entrained through the holes in the mask, thus diluting the total inhaled oxygen mixture. If the child takes a deeper breath, he or she entrains more air, and thus the inspired oxygen concentration falls. So, the concentration of inhaled oxygen varies with the tidal volume or peak inspiratory flow rate. Such masks are therefore classified as variable performance masks. The instruction leaflet that indicates the percentage oxygen at varying flow rates is, therefore, only an approximation (Table 9.2).

Table 9.2 Percentage oxygen at varying flow rates: Hudson mask (approximate)

Oxygen flow rate (l/min)	Oxygen concentration (%)
5	35
6	40
8	50

During expiration, some of the expired gas, containing CO_2, leaks out through the holes, preventing the accumulation of CO_2 – so called 're-breathing'. The amount of re-breathing is affected by the oxygen flow and the size of the mask – the reservoir.

Dual-prong nasal cannulae, or 'nasal specs', actually perform in a similar way to a variable performance mask. Instead of being the empty space inside the mask, the gas reservoir is the volume of the nasopharynx. Breathing in with the mouth closed will allow oxygen flow and some air entrainment through the nose. Breathing in with the mouth open would allow more air entrainment and dilute the inspired concentration of oxygen. The quoted inspired oxygen levels for nasal cannulae are of the same order as variable performance masks such as the Hudson mask (Table 9.3). Dry gas flows higher than 6 l/min are not well tolerated: they dry out the mucous membranes and promote upper airway irritation.

Table 9.3 Percentage oxygen at varying flow rates: 'nasal specs' (approximate)

Oxygen flow rate (l/min)	Oxygen concentration (%)
1	24
2	27
3	30
4	33
5	36
6	42

The efficiency of variable performance oxygen masks and 'nasal specs' depends on the tidal volume and the size of the reservoir. Masks are useful in children who are strictly mouth breathers, as well as some with extreme nasal irritation or epistaxis. On the negative side, masks are uncomfortable, confining, muffle communication and interfere with eating. 'Nasal specs' are generally much better tolerated in children; however, they should be correctly fitted and supervised.

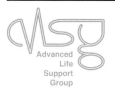

Non-re-breathing masks are fitted with a reservoir bag and a one-way valve to prevent mixing of expired gas with the reservoir gas. Oxygen flows into the reservoir bag at 8–10 l/min. When the child breathes in, the gas mixture from the mask is inhaled first, followed by gas from the reservoir bag. Provided that the reservoir bag is filled before use, and the mask is close fitting, there should be minimal air entrainment. Expired air containing CO_2 is vented through one-way valves built into the mask. Such devices, commonly called 'non rebreathing masks', are capable of delivering up to 90% oxygen (Figure 9.5).

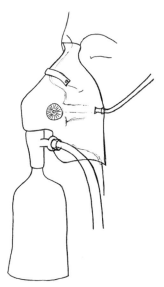

Fig. 9.5 Non rebreathing mask (with reservoir).

OXYGEN DELIVERY SYSTEMS

Anaesthetic circuits

These circuits require specific training for their proper use and must not be used by untrained individuals. It is also vital to note that a failure of the oxygen supply renders these circuits useless.

'Ayre's T-piece'

This breathing circuit is favoured by intensivists and anaesthetists, because it presents virtually no resistance to expiration and is able to deliver PEEP (positive end-expiratory pressure) and provide tactile feedback on the status of the child's lungs. It should be correctly referred to as a Jackson–Rees modification of an Ayre's T-piece or a Mapleson F breathing circuit (Figure 9.6). (An Ayre's T-piece is actually a Mapleson E configuration, which is not used – Figure 9.7.) The system is designed to be attached to a close-fitting facemask that is held in place over the child's nose and mouth to create a seal. The corrugated tube and open-ended bag act as a reservoir, filling with a mixture of exhaled and fresh gas during expiration and fresh gas during the expiratory phase. To prevent re-breathing, the fresh gas flow in a spontaneously breathing child must be maintained at two and a half to three times the child's minute volume. It is therefore suitable only for children up to about 25 kg in weight, above which a Mapleson C breathing circuit should be used.

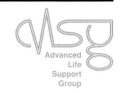

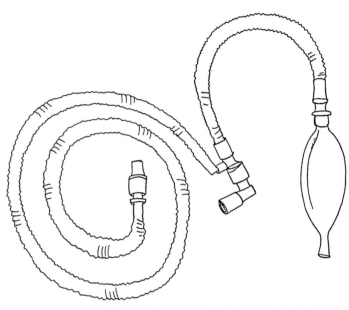

Fig. 9.6 The Jackson-Rees modified Ayre's T-piece (Mapleson F) circuit.

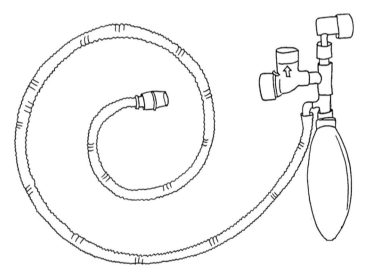

Fig. 9.7 The Mapleson C circuit.

Mapleson C circuit

In adults and older children weighing >25 kg a breathing circuit much used by anaesthetists is the Mapleson C or Water's circuit (Figure 9.8). As before, the system is designed to be attached to a close-fitting facemask that is held in place over the child's nose and mouth to create a seal. Oxygen is fed into the system between the reservoir bag and the spill valve, providing a large reservoir from which the child can breathe in. However, during expiration the expired gas containing CO_2 is mixed in the reservoir bag with incoming oxygen. As the bag distends, excess pressure is vented through an adjustable spill valve. There is great potential for re-breathing because, unlike the non-re-breathing masks described above, there is no one-way valve between the mask and the reservoir.

Increasing the oxygen flow rate to at least three times the child's spontaneous minute volume will minimise re-breathing and accumulation of CO_2. The Maple-

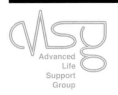

son C circuit allows the delivery of 100% oxygen and may be used manually to inflate the lungs by squeezing the reservoir bag. Failure of the oxygen supply renders the Mapleson C circuit useless.

> The self-inflating breathing circuit with one-way valve (and filter if needed) is a mandatory piece of transfer equipment for all circumstances

Self-inflating bag with one-way valve

The self-inflating breathing circuit is commonly referred to as a 'bag–valve–mask' or 'Ambu bag' (Figure 9.8). As with the anaesthetic circuits, the system enables the operator manually to inflate the lungs via a tight-fitting facemask to create a seal. The bag is made of silicone rubber, which, after squeezing, will re-expand as a result of its own elasticity. This means that the device can be used manually to inflate the lungs even in the absence of an oxygen supply. During spontaneous respiration, the child may inspire an oxygen-enriched gas mixture from the silicone bag. With the reservoir attached, it is possible to reach inspired oxygen concentrations of 90%. In the event of oxygen failure, air is entrained via a built-in valve. A bag–valve–mask system is not suitable for delivering oxygen to small, spontaneously breathing children.

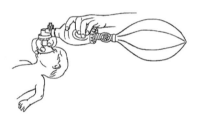

Fig. 9.8 Bag valve mask.

If they are not to be used for a single child, both the anaesthetic circuits and the self-inflating circuit should always be used with a bacterial filter placed between the circuit and the facemask.

All of the above circuits may also be used for manual ventilation of a child.

The ventilated child
Transport ventilators

Simple transport ventilators rely on oxygen pressure from the cylinder to drive the ventilator mechanics. Small transport ventilators, such as Babypac, Ventipac and Oxylog, use different volumes of oxygen depending on whether they are using 100% oxygen or entraining air. As a minimum the ventilator will consume the child's minute volume of oxygen when delivering 100%. Most ventilators will use at least an additional 1 l/min of oxygen as a 'driving gas' over and above that. When air is entrained, there may be some reduction in oxygen consumption; however, it is always prudent to plan the need for 100% oxygen.

Setting up paediatric ventilators is usually a matter of selecting a suitable peak inspiratory pressure, PEEP, inspiratory time and breath rate in order to achieve appropriate tidal and minute volumes. The inspired oxygen concentration may be titratable over a broad range (Babypac) or have two fixed values as provided by some older Oxylogs. The latter is also configured as a volume-limited machine and therefore must be either modified for use as a pressure-limited ventilator or used in its native mode. Volume-limited, time-cycled ventilation is extensively used in adult practice and is suitable for paediatric use in appropriately trained hands. Monitoring in basic models often involves no more than an airway pressure gauge. Alarms are often basic or even non-existent. Despite this, these ventilators are generally reliable and easy to use as they are robust and require no electricity as they are gas driven.

Advanced electronic circuitry in newer transport ventilators has enabled facilities, such as the ability of the ventilator to synchronise with the breathing efforts of non-paralysed children, to be incorporated. The display and alarm systems are more sophisticated but frequently not optimised for paediatric use. This technology requires electricity, and as a consequence these ventilators require a fully charged battery or mains supply.

> Formal training and education in the use of transport equipment is mandatory.

CALCULATING OXYGEN SUPPLIES

A simple oxygen consumption calculation should be made when planning the transportation of a child. First, ascertain what flow rate of oxygen is required to deliver appropriate ventilatory support, whether this is done using a mask, a breathing circuit or a ventilator. Always work on the basis of the worst-case scenario of deterioration. The journey time must then be estimated from its component parts (the transfer from the referring ward to the ambulance, the ambulance journey and the transfer from the ambulance to the receiving ward). For air transfers this sequence will occur twice, loading and unloading the aircraft (airport delays must also be considered).

It is important to plan for the worst-case scenario such as a major delay or a mechanical failure of the ventilator. Standard practice ensures that sufficient oxygen is carried to last for at least twice the anticipated journey time.

Spontaneous breathing and resuscitation circuits

The highest oxygen consumption by an oxygen mask is probably about $15 \, l/min$. This compares with the required flow rate for a non-re-breathing mask fitted with a reservoir bag, and the flow rate required for a breathing circuit.

> An O_2 consumption of $15 \, l/min$ is equivalent to $900 \, l/h$.

The ventilated child

A table on the ventilator or in the manufacturer's manual will detail the flow rate in l/min consumed by the ventilator for a given minute volume and inspiratory oxygen concentration. It should always be assumed that the child may need 100% oxygen. An allowance should also be made for deterioration en route that needs increased pressure. It should be noted that the driving gas has to be under some pressure (about 10bar) to enable the ventilator to function. Therefore, even though there may be some gas, under low pressure left in the cylinder, if the pressure falls below 10bar the ventilator will cease to function.

To calculate the required oxygen for a paediatric ventilator multiply the oxygen consumption in l/min by the length of the journey in minutes. For some

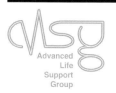

ventilators a flow rate is set that should be multiplied by the time for the journey. Once this figure is obtained, double it:

Oxygen requirement (l) = 2 × Ventilator consumption (l/min) × Total journey time (min).

To calculate what this means in terms of cylinders you need to know what each cylinder contains (see Table 9.4).

> Always add a safety factor to cope with delays, breakdowns, etc. At minimum, 'double up' the predicted gas supply.
> Always carry more than one cylinder in case one fails.

Table 9.4 Oxygen cylinder sizes and contents

Size of cylinder	Volume of gas (l)	Weight (kg) (full)	Height (cm)	Diameter (cm)	Valve	Aramid	Time (at 10 l/min)	Time (at 15 l/min)
C	170	2.23	490	89	Pin index	No	17 min	11 min
D	340	3.86	535	102	Pin index	No	34 min	22 min
CD[b]	460	3.25	480	100	Star Schräder	Yes	46 min	30 min
DD[a]	460	3.25	480	100	Star nipple	Yes	46 min	30 min
RD	460	4.65	480	100	Star Schräder	Yes	46 min	30 min
E	680	6.32	865	102	Pin index	No	68 min	44 min
F	1360	16.34	930	140	Bull nose	No	2 h 16 min	1 h 30 min
HX	2300	20.1	940	140	Star Schräder	Yes	3 h 50 min	2 h 33 min
ZX[c]	3040	14	940	143	Star Schräder	Yes	5 h 04 min	3 h 22 min

[a]DD cylinder Domiflow valve is restricted to 2–4 l flow – for the home market.
[b]See Figure 9.3.
[c]ZX cylinder is the same size as F and HX but contains more gas volume.
Calculated from data on BOC Gases website.

MONITORING THE CHILD

When contemplating the transfer of any child, either within a hospital or between different hospitals, the staff involved should consider how best to observe the child clinically for signs of deterioration. The usefulness of basic clinical observations involving the triad of look, listen and feel cannot be overestimated. Basic monitoring of airway, breathing and circulation (and in some children consciousness) must be undertaken intermittently during the most routine transfers, such as between an operating theatre and a ward.

Observations may be difficult during the transfer of a packaged critically ill child. However, they do form an essential starting point during the initial assessment and a fall-back position when more complex systems fail. Monitoring, via technology is fraught with problems. Clinical staff must understand how this monitoring works and its limitations.

Monitoring the airway

In the spontaneously breathing child this is undertaken simply by observing the ease with which he or she appears to be breathing. Look for signs of obstructed breathing – recession and tracheal tug – and listen for signs of obstruction, such as wheeze or stridor. In the ventilated child, close observations of chest movement, the airway pressure gauge and the capnograph should be used together with auscultation where appropriate.

Monitoring of oxygenation and respiration

The basic observations of looking for cyanosis and counting the respiratory rate in the spontaneously breathing child should not be forgotten. However, pulse oximetry is now widely available and capnography should be used during the transport of all ventilated children.

Pulse oximetry

This uses light absorption as a means of estimating arterial oxygen saturation. It is based on the fact that oxyhaemoglobin and deoxyhaemoglobin absorb visible red and invisible infrared electromagnetic radiation differently. The oximeter sends a light signal through a vascular bed, such as a finger or an earlobe, measures what is transmitted (or reflected), and then uses a number of algorithms to estimate the arterial oxygen saturation. As it is a mathematical prediction rather than a direct measurement, it is denoted as SpO_2 rather than SaO_2. Recent software developments such as Masimo's Signal Extraction Technology (SET) significantly reduce many of the problems associated with older pulse oximetry technology.

The accuracy of pulse oximetry

Pulse oximetry estimates the oxygen saturation of haemoglobin, which varies physiologically in accordance with the oxygen dissociation curve. This is sigmoid in shape and, at high arterial oxygen levels, flat. Consequently, it is often stated that oximetry is relatively insensitive at detecting hyperoxaemia in children with high baseline levels of measured oxygen tension in the blood (PaO_2). Essentially this means, in preterm babies, that a well-oxygenated child who has an SpO_2 of 100% may have a very high PaO_2.

As the SpO_2 falls to <90%, the accuracy becomes less, and with standard probes reading of less than 80% saturation should be viewed at best as a rough estimate. As a result of these inaccuracies, which occur not only between children but also within the same child over a period of time, it is considered good practice to compare an SpO_2 reading recorded at the same time as an arterial blood gas pO_2. As a result of higher levels of foetal haemoglobin, neonatal algorithms are neonate specific.

Masimo's SET equipment provides special probes that deliver improved accuracy at low oxygen concentrations.

Remember
- Oxygen saturation (SpO_2) is not the same as the pO_2 measured in arterial blood gases (PaO_2)
- In children an SpO_2 value in the high 80s may represent dangerously low values of PaO_2
- Although a high SpO_2 indicates that the blood is well oxygenated, it does not mean that the ventilation is adequate

---

Limitations of pulse oximetry

The theory of pulse oximetry and the relationship to the oxygen dissociation curve, is often poorly understood. Vasoconstriction, hypothermia and irregular

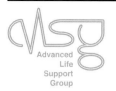

heart rhythms may make it difficult to detect a reliable signal from a pulse oximeter probe.

Movement and vibration artefacts can also result in unreliable readings. Such movement is inevitable during transportation. Masimo's SET oximeters have an enhanced ability to cope with vibration and vasoconstriction but are not infallible. Strong ambient light can contaminate the signal from the probe, although most machines can now compensate for this effect. Nail varnish, especially if blue, green or black, can cause inaccurate SpO_2 readings. Acrylic nails do not in themselves affect pulse oximetry, although long fingernails can impede positioning of the probe on the finger.

Intravenous dyes such as methylene blue and indocyanine green can falsely report low SpO_2 readings. Abnormal haemoglobinopathies may affect SpO_2 readings. High levels of carboxyhaemoglobin, which absorbs red light in a similar way to oxyhaemoglobin, may make the pulse oximeter overestimate the conventional SpO_2 reading.

Particular care should be taken in children with smoke inhalation injury and carbon monoxide poisoning. High methaemoglobin levels also interfere with the accuracy of the conventional SpO_2 readings, which tend to read 85%, regardless of the actual SaO_2.

Setting up and using the pulse oximeter

As with any medical device, the user should have received formal training in the use and care of the equipment:

- Switch on the monitor and wait for it to complete a system self-test.
- Select a probe that is compatible with the monitor, appropriate for the body part on which it is to be placed and suitable for the age and size of the child. Where possible use low-range probes if appropriate and available.
- Check that the probe is not damaged and secure it on the child (finger, earlobe or other body part, depending on the probe design).

Ensure that there is a good quality waveform before accepting the value of the SpO_2. If the machine does not have a waveform display, check the intensity scale as an alternative, but much less reliable, quality control signal. Check that the heart rate is registered on the pulse oximeter; it should agree with that from the ECG. If not, this may indicate an inadequate signal or machine error.

If the signal strength is low or the waveform is irregular, check that the probe is properly attached to the child. If the problem cannot be attributed to poor peripheral perfusion or movement artefact, check that the probe gives a good signal with a regular waveform and a normal reading when you place the probe on yourself. A low SpO_2 may reflect a problem with the child or with the monitor (measurement artefact). It is wise to assume that the problem lies with the child, but it is still important to check the waveform. Some causes of errors in pulse oximetry are listed in Box 9.1.

Box 9.1 Causes of errors in pulse oximetry

- Cold/hypovolaemia/vasoconstriction
- Movement/vibration
- NIBP (non-invasive blood pressure) cuff on the same arm
- Ambient light
- Unreliable under 85% saturation (75% in neonates) with standard probes
- Carboxyhaemoglobin/methaemoglobin

End-tidal CO₂ monitoring (capnography)

Capnography is the technique of measuring and displaying the carbon dioxide (CO_2) levels in the airway (Figure 9.9). CO_2 absorbs infrared radiation. During the respiratory cycle the CO_2 level in the respiratory gas is measured by comparing how much infrared radiation is absorbed in a sampling chamber compared with a known source. During inspiration (D–E) the level of CO_2 in the sampling chamber falls rapidly.

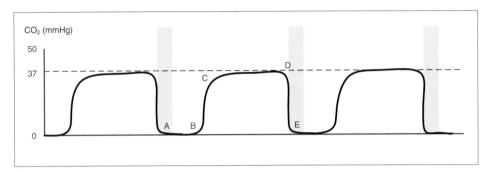

Fig. 9.9 The normal capnograph – grey shaded areas represent inspiration.

During A–B, the first part of expiration, dead space gas from the airway endotracheal tube, trachea, bronchi and bronchioles (down to, but not including, the respiratory bronchioles and alveoli) is exhaled first. The end-tidal CO_2 ($ETCO_2$) signal then rises (B–C) to a plateau (C–D), as the gas containing CO_2 from the alveoli and respiratory bronchioles is exhaled.

In healthy individuals, the CO_2 level at the end of expiration ($ETCO_2$) approximates the $PaCO_2$ (the partial pressure of CO_2 measured in arterial blood gases).

The capnometer provides valuable supplementary evidence that the endotracheal tube is in the correct position. If the tube has been dislodged into the oesophagus, it registers no or minimal CO_2. It can also be used to monitor respiratory rate and serves to indicate when a circuit disconnection has occurred.

There are two types of capnometer: sidestream and mainstream. The former sucks gas from the airway circuit through a fine-bore tube via a water trap and the sample is analysed within the machine itself; the latter's sensor is situated within the airway circuit. It does not require energy expenditure to suck up the gases but needs an electrical supply to the sensor itself. As a result, the mainstream sensor tends to be bulkier and more vulnerable to damage.

Setting up and using a capnometer

- All staff using the capnometer should be fully trained in its use.
- The capnometer should be calibrated at regular intervals according to the manufacturer's instructions.
- If using a mainstream capnometer, check that the sensor holder is patent and that the sensor panels are clean and not cracked.
- If using a sidestream capnometer, visually check the sampling tubing for signs of moisture and ensure that the water trap is empty.
- Switch on and allow a warm-up time with sensors attached to the breathing circuit.
- Ensure that the sensor or sampling tube is not lying lower than the endotracheal tube, so as to reduce the risk of secretions or condensation contaminating the sensor or blocking the tubing.

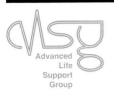

- Position the sensor or sampling tube to avoid traction on the endotracheal tube.
- Ensure that all airway connections are secure.

Limitations of capnometry

It is important not to regard the $ETCO_2$ value as an exact equivalent of the $PaCO_2$. In circumstances such as shock, the $ETCO_2$ is often less than the $PaCO_2$. This is a result of increased physiological dead space in the lungs caused by poor perfusion of upper (less dependent) parts of the lungs. The expired gas from these areas has a lower CO_2 concentration than from those areas that equilibrate well with blood flowing through the lungs. As a result, when the $ETCO_2$ is low, it remains uncertain whether the $PaCO_2$ is also low. There is no substitute for checking an arterial blood gas sample.

Correlating the $PaCO_2$ and the $ETCO_2$ before setting off on the journey is helpful in maintaining control en route, but great care must be taken in interpreting changes in the $ETCO_2$ if there are concomitant changes in the circulatory status (Box 9.2).

Box 9.2 Check the $ETCO_2$ against the $PaCO_2$

A reduced end-tidal CO_2 may be a result of hyperventilation or a ventilation/perfusion mismatch caused by:
- hypovolaemia
- sepsis
- heart failure
- pulmonary embolism

The $ETCO_2$ should be monitored in all intubated children. A high $ETCO_2$ generally indicates underventilation; if the $ETCO_2$ is 6 kPa (45 mmHg) in a child with normal lungs the ventilation may need to be increased.

A high $ETCO_2$ may relate to a problem with inadequate ventilator settings or to partial airway obstruction. Other causes include an increase in temperature or metabolic rate.

A falling $ETCO_2$ indicates overventilation or a fall in temperature or metabolic rate. The $ETCO_2$ may continue to slope upwards during late expiration, with loss of the plateau. This occurs when the airway or ventilator tubing becomes obstructed or bronchospasm develops. Excessive damping or flattening of the waveform may indicate blockage of the suction tubing in a sidestream capnometer. Contamination of a mainstream sensor by secretions may cause the $ETCO_2$ to be overestimated. High respiratory rates (>30/min) may preclude accurate measurement of $ETCO_2$, especially in sidestream capnometers. The fall in barometric pressure at an altitude can result in an underestimation of $ETCO_2$.

As in pulse oximetry, the waveform serves as a quality control signal from which to judge the reliability of the readings. If the function of the capnometer is in doubt, test it yourself, by exhaling into the sampling port to confirm a normal waveform with an expected $ETCO_2$ of 5.0–5.6 kPa (38–42 mmHg).

Monitoring the ventilated child during transportation

Monitoring of the ventilated child requires observeation of a number of individual components:
- The child's chest for signs of symmetrical movement, synchronous with the ventilator

- The child's breathing system connections
- The state of the oxygen supply
- The pulse oximeter display
- The capnography display
- The ventilator display, gauges and settings.

Monitoring the cardiovascular system

Basic observations are important during transfer of children. For short internal journeys basic observations can be quickly carried out to ensure that all is well, while waiting for a lift. The pulse can be assessed in terms of its rate, rhythm and quality, and the capillary refill time observed to mark peripheral perfusion. Over a longer period of time, the urine output is often a useful index of major organ perfusion.

The electrocardiogram

The electrocardiogram (ECG) is well established as a monitoring tool. It provides useful information about heart rate and arrhythmias. For acute episodes of hypoxia, bradycardia in babies may act as a backup alarm.

Effective monitoring and the interpretation of the ECG trace during the transfer of any child may be made difficult by artefacts. Despite the use of modern artefact-rejection monitors, problems are often encountered. High-frequency filters reduce distortions from muscle movement, mains current and electromagnetic interference from other equipment. The low-frequency filters reduce respiratory and transfer induced body movement artefact. However, the reliance on the smart monitor has possibly led to a reduction in the care with which children are monitored. In neonates leads are frequently displaced.

The silver/chloride electrodes need to have the best possible electrical connection between the electrode and the skin. The correct storage of electrodes is vitally important; the conducting gel must not be allowed to dry out. Placing electrodes over bony prominences will reduce artefact from muscle movement.

Shielding of cables and leads helps to reduce interference from AC mains and radiofrequency-induced currents. This shielding consists of electroconductive woven material that is 'earthed'; any interference currents are induced in the metal screen and not in the monitoring leads. However, the 'flying leads' leading to the electrodes have much less shielding. It is therefore good practice to prevent these leads from moving, especially during transfer; a hypoallergenic tape can be used to strap them on to the child's chest.

> Careful attention paid to electrode storage and application will help to reduce ECG artefact.

Blood pressure measurement

Non-invasive blood pressure (NIBP) measurement has a role in the intrahospital transportation of non-critically ill children. However, in interhospital transport medicine, the major disadvantages include motion artefact and the rapid depletion of battery power as a result of the pneumatic pump's power consumption. Invasive arterial and central venous pressure (CVP) monitoring are recommended for the transportation of critically ill children. NIBP may be considered as a backup system.

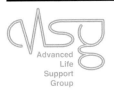

Invasive arterial pressure monitoring

Arterial pressure may be conveniently measured on a beat-to-beat basis using an intra-arterial cannula attached to a transducer. The transducer converts the physical pressure wave into an electrical signal which is amplified and displayed by the monitor. Intra-arterial lines should be continually flushed at 0.5–2 ml/h with heparinised saline, delivered by syringe driver or pressure bag system.

Clinical problems

It is important to remember that a normal blood pressure does not necessarily indicate adequate cardiac output. The waveform may indicate clinical problems; a spiky waveform with a short systolic time may be seen in hypovolaemia. Further, an arterial trace that seems to swing with respiration is associated with hypovolaemia – so-called 'pre-load responsiveness'. Some monitors will measure this variation and deliver a figure for pulse pressure variation. The waveform may also reveal technical problems, such as a resonant, overshooting trace or a flattened, over-damped trace. In such cases it is worth rechecking for bubbles and leaks and to flush the line manually. Consider removing any unnecessary three-way taps or excessive tubing. Consider re-zeroing and comparing the readings with NIBP values in the event of unexpected values, but do not simply ascribe abnormalities to monitor dysfunction. It is more likely that the fault lies with the child, who may need urgent attention. Re-zero periodically during prolonged transfers.

Invasive CVP monitoring

With the advent of central venous catheters made up of multiple lumina, some might argue that there is less need for large-bore peripheral lines; however, central venous lines can become dislodged, thus losing one or all lumina. You should work on the basis that the worst-case scenario occurs – the line extravasates.

Monitoring the nervous system

Basic clinical skills involving close observation of the child's reaction to stimuli and compliance with treatment form the mainstay of neurological monitoring. In the conscious child this is not difficult. However, many critically ill children undergoing transportation are sedated and paralysed. The clinician is therefore reliant on surrogate measures of awareness and pain such as pulse rate, blood pressure and the presence of sweating. Pupil size and reaction are especially relevant in the brain-injured child.

POWER SUPPLIES: BATTERIES AND INVERTERS

Reports of critical care equipment failure during transfer occur with frightening regularity. Many of these are the result of battery failure. Staff involved in transfer medicine rely on power supplies almost as much as they do on oxygen. There are two types of battery in current use: rechargeable and non-rechargeable (Table 9.5).

Table 9.5 Common types of batteries

Type	Construction
Non-rechargeable	Zinc carbon, zinc chloride and alkaline batteries
Rechargeable	Nickel cadmium (NiCd), nickel metal hydride (NiMH), lithium (Li) ion and sealed lead acid (SLA)

One of the most important observed differences between non-rechargeable and rechargeable batteries is the discharge characteristics. Figure 9.10 contrasts a non-rechargeable alkaline battery with a rechargeable NiCd battery. The alkaline battery power output deteriorates slowly, whereas the NiCd battery loses power over a few minutes.

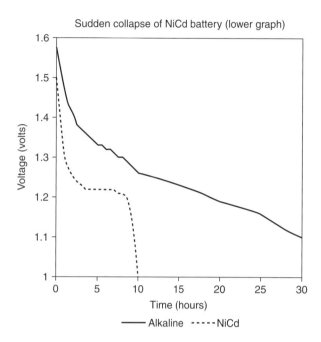

Fig. 9.10 Discharge curves for AA size batteries: in both cases the discharge current is 60 mA. Contrasts between a non-rechargeable alkaline battery and a rechargeable NiCd battery. (Reproduced with permission from Medical Devices Agency.)

In general, rechargeable batteries do not store as much energy as non-rechargeable batteries; however, sealed lead acid batteries are used in some heavy-duty applications (Table 9.6).

Table 9.6 Common uses for rechargeable batteries

Construction	Uses
Nickel cadmium (NiCd)	Cell phones, video cameras, many syringe drivers
Nickel metal hydride (NiMH)	Mobile phones and laptops
Sealed lead acid (SLA)	Heavy applications:
	Defibrillators
	Mobile X-ray machines
	Wheelchairs
	UPS systems

UPS, uninterruptible power supply.

NiCd batteries, which have a wide range of applications in medical devices, have the shortest charging time, but are demanding on 'exercise requirements'. This means that if the periodic discharge cycle is omitted the battery loses performance as a result of crystalline formation. When this premature ageing of the battery pack occurs, although 'fully charged', the battery eventually regresses to a point where it can hold less than half of its original capacity, even after charging. This will result in unexpected battery failure.

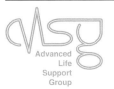

Many biomedical devices such as syringe drivers have built-in battery management systems that will automatically recharge the battery when necessary, generally while allowing the device to continue working on AC mains. However, if the battery becomes completely flat during a transfer, the operation of the internal power supply fails first and, consequently, a syringe driver may appear to be working, but there is not enough power to run the alarm function. There is no warning when the pump suddenly stops. A number of syringe driver manufacturers have stopped promoting their battery backup as reliable for the transfer environment.

> - NiCd batteries usually need exercising by periodically fully discharging
> - Implement the manufacturer's instructions about charging and discharging batteries
> - Be aware that rechargeable batteries fail very quickly.

If you suspect that the equipment is not working correctly, or there has been a battery failure, make sure that the equipment is taken out of service and sent to a biomedical engineer for a battery function check. It is helpful to describe to the engineer the exact circumstances of the failure.

Modern ambulances have some spare capacity in their battery systems and it is possible to convert the battery's 12 V DC into 240 V AC. This requires an inverter that may be connected to the incubator terminals of the ambulance's power supply. Before purchasing or using an inverter, the practicalities must be discussed with the ambulance service and its autoelectrical team.

SUMMARY

An understanding of the calculation of oxygen requirements and different oxygen delivery systems is essential for safe transfer. Clinical monitoring can be helpful for short transfers but generally will be supplemented by electronic monitoring often of multiple parameters.

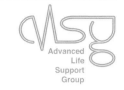

CHAPTER 10

Securing and packaging

LEARNING OBJECTIVES

In this chapter you will learn about:
- The concepts of security, accessibility and thermoregulation in relation to:
  Endotracheal tubes
  Intravascular lines
  Chest drains
  Equipment

SECURITY AND ACCESSIBILITY

Securing endotracheal tubes

ET tubes are at risk of being dislodged unless they are secured adequately. Neonatal ET tubes are often fixed using proprietary clip systems. Otherwise, the preferred method of securing ET tubes in children uses adhesive tape as described below. The cotton-tape methodology used in intubated adults is not recommended in children.

Securing a paediatric nasotracheal tube with adhesive tape
The Melbourne strapping technique

To prevent skin damage caused by adhesive tape, the child's skin should be protected with a proprietary skin protecting adhesive dressing such as DuoDERM. Such dressings consist of a flexible, polyurethane, outer foam layer and an adhesive, skin contact layer that contains a moisture-absorbing hydrocolloid material.

The taping procedure is classically described for nasal intubation and comprises the use of three separate pieces of adhesive tape. The application procedure is described below.

Melbourne strapping procedure

1 Cut a length of string slightly longer than the distance around the child's face from one ear to the other.
2 Tie the string around the ET tube with a single knot positioned posteriorly. The tube may then be held securely in place by an assistant holding the string (Figure 10.1).

Paediatric and Neonatal Safe Transfer and Retrieval: The Practical Approach, Edited by Steve Byrne, Steve Fisher, Peter-Marc Fortune, Cassie Lawn and Sue Wieteska. © 2008 Blackwell Publishing, ISBN: 978-1-4051-6919-6.

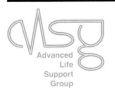

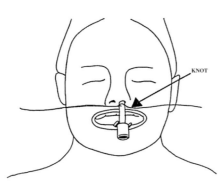

Fig. 10.1 Tie string around tube.

3 Prepare skin-protecting patches (Figure 10.2): to affix directly to facial skin as shown, use DuoDERM or equivalent.

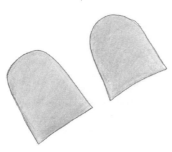

Fig. 10.2 Prepare DuoDERM skin protecting patches.

4 Use strips of Sleek or Elastoplast to prepare two 'trouser legs' and one 'eye hole'. The trouser legs need to be long enough to pass across the nose and wrap around the ET tube. Each trouser leg must have a thick and a thin limb (Figure 10.3).

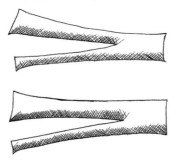

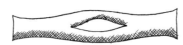

Fig. 10.3 Adhesive tape preparation: two trouser legs and one eye hole.

5 Place DuoDERM patches on the face on either side of nose to protect the skin (under the string – Figure 10.4).

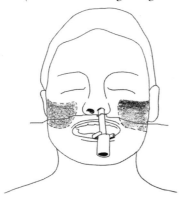

Fig. 10.4 Application of DuoDERM skin protection patches.

6 Place the wide part of first trouser leg over the stretched string, on the side of face furthest from the ET tube. Apply the inferior leg of the trouser under the nose and on to DuoDERM on the other side (Figure 10.5).

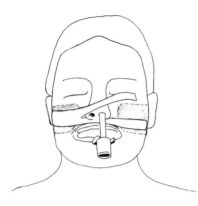

Fig. 10.5 Application of first trouser leg: inferior leg under nose.

7 Stretch and apply superior trouser leg over the nose and around the ET tube. The tape should pass from nose to tube at the lateral edge of the nares as shown (Figure 10.6).

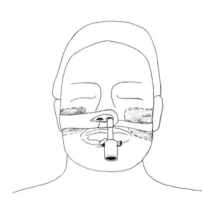

Fig. 10.6 Application of first trouser leg: superior leg wrapped around endotracheal tube.

8 Repeat the same procedure starting with the wide part of second trouser leg, passing from the same side as the ET tube. On this occasion the superior leg passes over the nose and on to the opposite cheek (Figure 10.7).

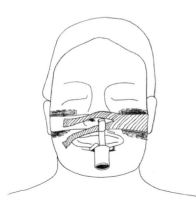

Fig. 10.7 Application of second trouser leg: superior leg over nose.

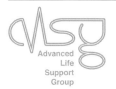

9 The inferior leg is stretched up and around the ET tube, from below (Figure 10.8).

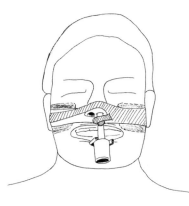

Fig. 10.8 Application of second trouser leg: inferior leg wrapped around endotracheal tube.

10 Place the 'eye hole' over previous tapes, ensuring that the maximum visibility of skin surface around both nostrils is achieved. Note that the application is most easily achieved by removing the ET tube connector to prevent catching.

11 Finally, replace the ET tube connector (Figure 10.9).

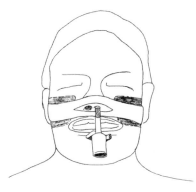

Fig. 10.9 Completed Melbourne strapping.

12 On completion most of the circumference of the intubated nostril should remain visible for inspection.

Securing intravascular lines

All intravenous and arterial lines must be adequately secured before transfer. They can be easily dislodged during movement between the bed/cot and stretcher, into and out of an incubator, in and out of the vehicle, and through use within the confines of a moving ambulance if they are not well secured and protected. The same concepts apply to securing intravenous lines for a child before computed tomography (CT).

Peripheral intravenous cannulae should be fixed in place with commercially available adhesive dressings or non-allergenic adhesive tape applied to dry skin. Dressings that cover the entry point of the cannula must be transparent and should be regularly inspected for signs of extravasation. Bandages that completely cover the cannula must not be used. Infusion tubing connected to the cannula should be secured by taping a loop of tubing to the child; this helps to prevent pulling and accidental removal of the cannula. Central venous lines should be stitched in place after insertion (except in the extreme preterm baby). The insertion sites should be covered with a transparent, adhesive dressing. Adequate lengths of infusion tubing are needed in order to prevent excessive tension on the cannula. All connections must be Luer locked to minimise the risk of accidental disconnection.

Two intravenous access points for administration of fluids and medications should be considered the minimum number required for a transfer. In a shocked child one or both of these access routes may have to be intraosseous. It is important to preserve the function of the latter by attaching extension tubing. This minimises movements at the point where the needle punctures the bone. Even small lateral movements can rapidly lead to mechanical failure and extravasation. The intraosseous needle should be supported perpendicular to the limb. This may be achieved using cut gauze and tapes as shown in Figure 10.10 and 10.11. There is some evidence that IO needles inserted using proprietary devices such as EZ-IO or bone injection gun (BIG) are less prone to displacement.

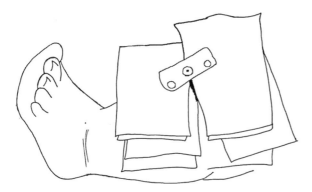

Fig. 10.10 Cut gauze and tapes.

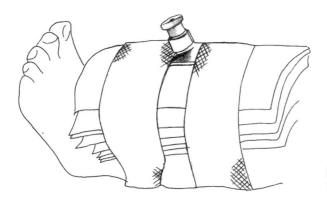

Fig. 10.11 Securing of an intraosseous line.

> Intravascular lines are vulnerable to accidental displacement during transport. Particular care should be taken to ensure that excessive strains are not placed on the lines and connections.

Securing chest drains

Chest drains should be secured to minimise the risk of dislodgement. A chest drain that falls out in a ventilated child may rapidly lead to the recurrence of a pneumothorax.

Procedure for securing a chest drain

1 To secure the drain, a suture should be used. Neonatal drains may be held in place with Steri-Strips and clear adhesive dressing rather than sutures, according to local practice.

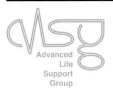

2 Pass the suture through both skin and subcutaneous tissue of sufficient bulk to afford a good purchase.
3 Tie a locking knot.
4 Pass both ends of the suture behind the chest drain and bring them to the front.
5 Tie a locking knot.

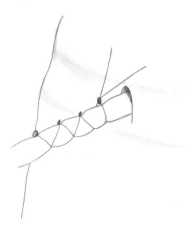

Fig. 10.12 Suturing a chest drain.

6 Pass both ends of the suture around the drain again and bring to the front.
7 Tie another locking knot.
8 Repeat steps 7 and 8 several times, making a criss-cross pattern along the drain.
9 Note that when tying the locking knots, try to indent the drain gently with the suture without snapping it (Figure 10.12)

Steps 5–9 may be replaced by tying the suture through a proprietary tube clip system (Figure 10.13).

(a) Front view   (b) Lateral view (closeup)

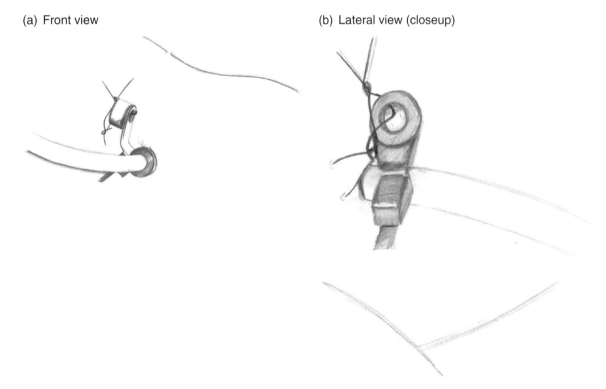

Fig. 10.13 Securing a chest drain with proprietary tube clip system.

STABLE, SECURE EQUIPMENT POSITIONING AND THERMOREGULATION

Having secured the ET tube, intravascular lines, chest drains and catheters to the child, attention must be turned to packaging them in a way that provides security as well as accessibility. The transfer team should consider the mode of transport (hospital trolley, ambulance or aircraft), and all monitoring and supporting equipment when formulating their packaging plans. Transfer to the CT or MR (magnetic resonance) scanner should be planned with knowledge of the layout of the scanning room.

Plan ahead; ensure that from a secure seat in the vehicle, members of the team will have visual and tactile access to the child. Most UK ambulances are configured as shown in Figure 10.14.

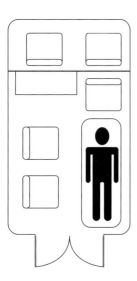

Fig. 10.14 Common UK ambulance layout.

Access to intravascular lines or pressure transducers placed on the child's left-hand side may be almost impossible from any seated position. Where possible, plan to secure these to the child's right-hand side. This may be best achieved using an intravenous extension with a three-way tap in-line. Urine drainage bags and chest drains are also safer and more accessible when secured to the stretcher on the child's right side.

The ABCDE approach should be used when packaging the child. Ensure that all airway and breathing system connections are correctly and firmly joined. Check the high-pressure oxygen and air connections to the ventilator, because a leak from this part of the system can rapidly drain cylinders. A secondary manual circuit to support ventilation should be attached to an independent oxygen supply for emergency use. Suctioning the ET tube during the transfer may be easier and safer using a closed-suction device. Any items for use during the transfer also require securing, such as pre-filled syringes, suction tubing and reintubation equipment. These should be in closed containers/bags and safely secured to ensure that they do not endanger anyone in case of a crash.

Cables, and intravascular lines, are usually tidier and easier to handle if bundled together using proprietary cable tidies or, alternatively, split 22 mm ventilator tubing; the secret is to use a number of short (5 cm) sections, rather than one long length. Labelling any lines with the name of the drug being infused will reduce the risk of inadvertently flushing a bolus of an incorrect drug, particularly

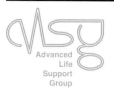

inotropic agents. All equipment such as the transport ventilator and syringe pumps must be secured (see Chapter 17).

Protect the eyes of unconscious and muscle-relaxed children, by closing with Geliperm or similar. This may be easily removed during the transfer to check the pupils. The use of head blocks or sandbags is mandatory in all children who have sustained traumatic injuries and whose cervical spine has not been 'cleared'. They may also be used in any sedated, muscle-relaxed and ventilated child to add stability to the head and neck, preventing side-to-side movement, which will have an adverse effect on ET tube security. In addition this central alignment of the head in the unconscious child optimises cerebral venous return. Many transport teams use a vacuum mattress that may be moulded to the child just before starting transfer for this purpose (see Figure 6.2).

> Use head blocks or a vacuum mattress to stabilise an unconscious, intubated child for transfer.

The actual process of wrapping the child can be varied according to the child's size, clinical condition and the resources available. Sheets, blankets, hat, socks, mittens, space blanket or bubble wrap may all be used as appropriate. To allow optimal visualisation and reduce heat loss, bubble wrap may be used for babies, with the entire length of an intubated baby being covered, to maintain thermal control. If heat loss or climate influences are an issue, a chemical gel-warming pad, such as a Transwarmer mattress, may be used. By activating the gel to create a chemical reaction, the latent heat of crystallisation will generate heat for several hours. These mattresses are safe and effective only if they are activated from an initial temperature of 19–28°C because they generate a set amount of heat. Activating them when they are too hot or too cold risks burning or cooling the child. Also, when using warming pads on sedated and muscle-relaxed children, the skin must be monitored to prevent any thermal injury occurring. Insulating the head, particularly in infants, will significantly reduce heat loss; this can be achieved with a hat/bonnet or any readily available dressings such as Tubigauze or Gamgee.

Moving the sedated and intubated child from a bed to a stretcher or vice versa can be difficult, even with handling aids such as the Patslide. Some transfers involve secondary moves before the final destination (for example, into a CT scanner or helicopter).

Some children, who have suffered major trauma or spinal injuries, they may be easier to handle when placed on a long spinal board. However, poor tissue perfusion of dependent areas and the use of spinal boards can result in pressure sores, so the time spent on the spinal board should be kept to a minimum.

The use of a vacuum mattress will improve the security and immobilisation of children of all ages. The mattress is suctioned via the integral valve, which creates a vacuum around the internal beads, turning the flexible mattress into a firm, moulded support. These mattresses may have straps to secure the child, and side-carrying handles enabling moving them with minimal handling.

Securing smaller children – that is, pre-school age – has been improved with devices such as the Pedi-Mate which harnesses around the child, with a five-point harness, and has straps to secure it to the ambulance stretcher. Any such securing devices should be specifically tested to CEN standards (see Chapter 17). A new commercially available neonatal restraint, the neorestraint, is now available.

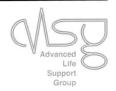

Finally, to conclude the packaging of the child:

- Check that the ET tube, intravascular lines, drains and transducers are secure
- Fasten the monitor cables together where possible
- Ensure easy access to at least one intravenous access point for use during transfer
- Protect and stabilise the child
- Fasten all the securing straps
- Plan thermoregulation; consider insulating the head
- Ensure easy access to resources for emergency interventions during transfer.

Once wrapped, the child should not be exposed again unless absolutely necessary.

SUMMARY

Close attention to security, accessibility and thermoregulation when securing and packaging a child will minimise the risk of adverse events and optimise the child's physiological status during transfer.

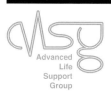

PART IV

Assessment and clinical aspects of transfer medicine

INTRODUCTION

The previous sections of this book have described the general principles of ACCEPT which can be applied to any transfer situation.

The Paediatric and Neonatal Safe Transfer and Retrieval course has to assume that the participants have some clinical knowledge and experience. The following chapters may be used as a reminder of the key principles involved in the assessment and initial stabilisation of children prior to transfer; readers may also find the pages within this section a useful reference when planning specific transfers.

Chapter 11 describes, in some detail, the concepts of primary and secondary surveys. Within the primary survey section, the ABCDE approach to the clinical assessment of children is accompanied by notes which may help the less experienced practitioner to understand the physiology behind the assessment and treatment of common clinical problems. For each of the major systems, specific examples of clinical problems are discussed. The use of primary and secondary surveys has more readily recognisable relevance to paediatric resuscitation and stabilisation than to neonatal. However it can usefully be applied to neonatal practice; the special issues that occur around the time of birth are highlighted in this chapter.

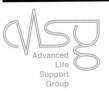

CHAPTER 11

Introduction to the clinical assessment of children

LEARNING OBJECTIVES

In this chapter you will learn about:

- The structured clinical approach to the assessment and initial care of a child requiring transfer, combining the use of primary and secondary surveys with the ABCDE approach
- The use of simple clinical assessment skills before proceeding to more complex methods of assessment
- The specific conditions that may need to be considered in the newborn

---

INTRODUCTION

The ABCDE approach, used to describe the sequence of the assessment and care of airway, breathing and circulation systems, was first developed in the United States in the 1970s as part of the then new Advanced Life Support (ALS) system of education. This alphabetical approach is now well established worldwide and has been extended by individual clinical groups (Box 11.1).

Box 11.1 The ABCDE approach

A   Airway assessment and control
B   Breathing
C   Circulation
D   Disability
E   Exposure (including temperature)

PRIMARY AND SECONDARY SURVEYS

The aim of the primary survey is to identify and treat any immediately life threatening conditions. The assessment process will obviously take into account the history of events leading up to the referral, a physical examination, followed by initial treatment. During the primary survey, arrangements should be made to commence monitoring of the child. This will establish a baseline. Changes in the

---

Paediatric and Neonatal Safe Transfer and Retrieval: The Practical Approach, Edited by Steve Byrne, Steve Fisher, Peter-Marc Fortune, Cassie Lawn and Sue Wieteska. © 2008 Blackwell Publishing, ISBN: 978-1-4051-6919-6.

child's clinical condition may then be tracked (Box 11.2). If the child's condition deteriorates at any stage the primary assessment must be repeated, starting with A.

The aim of the secondary survey is to systematically examine the child and identify problems which are significant but not immediately life threatening.

> Primary and secondary surveys can be applied to both paediatric and neonatal cases.

Box 11.2 Monitoring vital signs starts during the primary survey

- Respiratory rate
- Peripheral oxygen saturation
- Heart rate
- Blood pressure
- Pulse pressure
- Capillary refill
- Chest leads (ECG rhythm and waveform)
- Temperature (core and peripheral)

Primary survey

The aim of the primary survey is to identify and treat any immediately life-threatening conditions. This differs from the traditional clinical teaching, i.e. taking a history followed by clinical examination. This ensures that there are no delays in implementing life-saving treatment.

Box 11.3 Key components of the primary survey are:

Airway
Breathing
Circulation (and initial haemorrhage control when appropriate)
Disability
Exposure (including temperature)

Once any immediately life-threatening conditions have been either treated or excluded, a comprehensive history can be taken and a thorough examination carried out. This is known as the secondary survey and is dealt with later in this chapter. During this phase emergency treatment should continue as necessary. By the end of the secondary survey a formal management plan must be developed. This needs to include consideration of whether the child requires transportation to another facility.

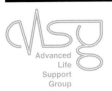

> **Primary survey**
> Rapidly seek out and treat all immediately life-threatening conditions.

The secondary survey

During the secondary survey the aim is to find new features and corroborative evidence to support, or refute, the working diagnosis and formulate plans for ongoing investigation and treatment, which will include decisions about the best location to continue this care. The key components are:

- A detailed medical history
- A full examination
- Appropriate investigations
- Formulation of a definitive plan for continuing care

THE PRIMARY AND SECONDARY SURVEY IN PRACTICE

Children who are in transit between referring and receiving centres should, where possible, be fully resuscitated and stable before departure. They may require care modalities not available in the referring unit. The need for active resuscitation and stabilisation during transfer should be the exception. A systematic approach to rapid clinical assessment, for use both prior to departure and during transfer, is extremely useful.

A B – Airway and Breathing

Respiratory decompensation in children can be rapid especially in infants. This is because of anatomical and physiological features that are unique to this group. These features may be particularly pronounced in newborn and preterm infants. They are listed in Table 11.1. Emboldened features may all make intubation more difficult.

Oxygen consumption in the newborn (7 ml/kg/min) is approximately twice that in adults. The gas available for exchange at alveolar level (alveolar ventilation) is the difference between the total minute ventilation and the dead space ventilation. In other words:

Alveolar ventilation = Respiratory rate × (Tidal volume − Dead space volume).

Infants have a relative inability to easily increase their tidal volumes. This is because they have a compliant ribcage and this may be exacerbated by stiff lungs (for example, in surfactant deficiency). Therefore respiratory distress is often an early sign of physiological stress in the infant. For example, tachypnoea may develop, to increase minute ventilation, in response to metabolic acidosis with or without raised CO_2 levels.

As dead space is usually constant, inadequate gas for exchange at alveolar level arises from reduction in tidal volumes or respiratory rate. This may occur as a result of either pulmonary pathology or reduced effort as the child tires. Newborns also have a relatively low functional residual capacity (FRC), which is the volume of gas left in the lungs at the end of normal tidal expiration. This gas acts as a reservoir for oxygen and prevents alveolar collapse. The reduction in FRC may be further exacerbated in respiratory diseases such as hyaline membrane disease or pneumonia. Grunting (forced expirations against a partially closed glottis) increases FRC and helps recruit alveoli.

Table 11.1 Anatomical differences between infants and children

Anatomy	Effect on airway/breathing
Large occiput	↑ neck flexion potentially causing airway obstruction
Large tongue	↑ risk of airway obstruction
Floppy epiglottis	↑ risk of airway obstruction
Larynx anterior/cephalad	
Short trachea	
Trachea angled posteriorly	
Low pharyngeal muscle tone	↑ risk of airway obstruction
Small nares	↑ airway resistance (<3 months usually nasal breathers)
Cricoid cartilage	Narrowest point up to 8 years
Narrow airways	↑ airway resistance
Compliant airways	May collapse with increased respiratory effort
Compliant chest wall	Inefficient delivery of respiratory muscle effort
Barrel shaped chest	Horizontal ribs reduce the contribution of chest wall movement to lung inflation
Flattened diaphragm	Reduced diaphragmatic movement
Immature respiratory muscles	Reduced effectiveness of forced expiration, for example, cough

Printed with kind permission from Paediatric and Neonatal Critical Care Transport, BMJ Books 2003.

Intercostal, subcostal, supraclavicular and sternal retractions result from increased muscle effort, in the presence of a compliant chest wall, to maintain adequate ventilation. Nasal flaring signals a child's effort to maximise air entry through the nose by minimising upper airway resistance.

Children must always be examined for signs of airway or breathing compromise. The patency of the airway and effectiveness of respiration can be assessed by looking, listening and feeling.

- Look:
  - cyanosis, pallor
  - chest movement – adequacy and symmetry
  - intercostal/subcostal/sternal recession and suprasternal retraction
  - head bob, nasal flare
  - apnoeas
  - ET tube size/patency/fixation
  - inspired oxygen requirement – trend
  - blood gas results
  - transilluminate the chest for a pneumothorax (check chest radiograph if available)
- Listen:
  - grunting
  - stridor
  - breath sounds: present/equal, for synchrony with ventilator if ventilated
- Feel:
  - expired air
  - chest movement
  - trapped secretions.

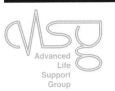

The immediate management of life-threatening respiratory problems

The primary survey treatment should include:

- Securing a patent airway: consider airway adjuncts such as a Guedel or naso-pharyngeal airway – intubation may be necessary.
- Administering oxygen.

A definitive decision must then be taken on the need for intubation either to secure the airway or to support adequate oxygenation and ventilation.

Intubation

Consider intubation and ventilation if the child:

- is unstable
- is not protecting their airway
- has a rapidly rising oxygen requirement or a requirement in excess of 50%
- is struggling to breathe or tiring (recession, grunting, head bobbing, tracheal tug)
- has rising PCO_2
- has recurrent apnoeas
- is <30 weeks' gestation.

Pneumothorax

A high index of suspicion about the possibility of a pneumothorax should be maintained in children with respiratory compromise, especially after sudden deterioration. Infants with possible hyaline membrane disease or children requiring high ventilator pressures are at particular risk.

Children who have developed a tension pneumothorax become progressively more difficult to ventilate as the intrapleural pressure increases. They may rapidly develop shock, as their cardiac output (CO) falls as a result of obstruction to venous return. Diagnosis of a tension pneumothorax must be made on clinical grounds because a child can arrest and potentially die in the time that it takes to obtain a chest radiograph.

If a tension pneumothorax has been diagnosed a 21 or 23 G butterfly or cannula attached to a three-way tap should be inserted into the second intercostal space in the midclavicular line on the side of tension. The air may then escape via the tap. This procedure provides temporary chest drainage and a definitive chest drain will need to be sited as a matter of urgency.

Note that, if no pneumothorax was present, the passage of the needle will increase the risk that one has been created. An urgent chest radiograph must always be performed in these circumstances.

Circulation

The aim of the primary cardiovascular survey is to detect whether the circulation is able to supply the tissues with adequate oxygen and remove the waste products of metabolism. Failure to do this is described as shock. Adequate oxygen delivery to the tissues requires a sufficient CO *and* a sufficient blood oxygen content. Oxygen is predominantly carried in red blood cells as oxyhaemoglobin. Therefore significant anaemia may result in a more rapid onset of shock as CO decreases. Significant polycythaemia makes the blood more viscous. This may reduce tissue perfusion and consequently oxygen delivery and may worsen pre-existing pulmonary hypertension.

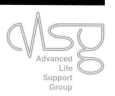

Cardiac output

Cardiac output is the amount of blood pumped into the circulation:

CO = Heart rate (HR) × Stroke volume (SV).

The stroke volume is determined by how well the ventricle fills during diastole and its ability to pump blood forward during systole. Consequently it is affected by, and may be manipulated through, changes in preload, contractility and afterload. It is important to note that leaky heart valves may result in back flow, reducing effective CO.

The newborn myocardium is less compliant than that of the older child. It is therefore less tolerant of increases in afterload and less responsive to increases in preload than older children and adults. In other words, infants are less able than adults to vary their stroke volume. They are consequently more dependent on increasing their heart rate to increase their CO. This is especially so in the preterm infant.

Preload

Preload refers to the volume of blood that flows into the heart during diastole. A reduction in preload reduces stroke volume. This may commonly occur secondary to hypovolaemia, causing reduced venous return and filling. Raised intrathoracic pressures may also reduce venous return. This may occur secondary to a tension pneumothorax or positive pressure ventilation. In rare circumstances a cardiac tamponade may directly reduce filling of the heart. Severe tachycardias may also result in such short periods of diastole that the heart is unable to fill adequately.

Hypovolaemia may result from the following:
- High fluid loss/'third spacing': for example, with necrotising enterocolitis/burns
- Sepsis: causing capillary leak and poor vascular tone
- Anaphylaxis: poor vascular tone (functional hypovolaemia)

Contractility

Contractility is a measure of the shortening ability of the cardiac muscle fibres. This describes the effectiveness of the pumping ability of the heart. Poor contractility reduces CO and is associated with:
- hypoxia
- hypoglycaemia
- sepsis (for example, group B streptococcal infection)
- some types of congenital heart disease
- hydrops foetalis
- myocarditis
- hypocalcaemia
- abnormal cardiac conduction.

Afterload

This is the pressure against which the ventricles must pump to eject blood. Constricted arterial blood vessels in both the peripheral and pulmonary circulations increase afterload and reduce CO. Increased afterload in obstructive congenital cardiac lesions, such as aortic stenosis or coarctation of the aorta, can lead to reduced CO and may rapidly lead to cardiac failure.

Blood pressure (Table 11.2)

Blood pressure is often used as a surrogate measure for adequate CO. This is potentially dangerous because it does not account for the influence of the child's

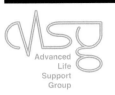

Table 11.2 Mean blood pressure and heart rate by age (for pre-term see Table 11.3)

Age (years)	Mean blood pressure (mmHg)	Heart rate
1 mth–1 yr	45–90	95–175
1–2	50–100	110–175
2–5	50–100	80–140
5–12	60–95	60–120
>12	65–100	60–100

peripheral vascular tone. In some disease states, normal regulation of vascular tone that ensures adequate blood supply to the brain, heart and kidneys may be dysfunctional. However, in most situations maintenance of an adequate blood pressure will usually ensure that the vital organs are adequately perfused. A good clinical sign may be drawn from observing the child's urine output. In the absence of renal disease or high blood osmolality (diabetic ketoacidosis or DKA), an output of 1–2 ml/kg/h suggests that the kidneys are adequately perfused. This can be particularly useful when blood pressure is borderline. Acid–base balance may also be monitored in this regard, because low output states will usually be reflected by a metabolic acidosis.

Septic shock
Children with sepsis are often initially peripherally shut down in an effort to maintain their blood pressure. This may mask a reduced, possibly inadequate, CO. Some children may present with reduced peripheral vascular tone (warm shock). Furthermore, as sepsis progresses, children who were initially peripherally shut down may lose homeostatic control. Vasodilatation results and loss of the integrity of the microvascular system may cause a reduction in venous return. This reduces preload and therefore CO, and ultimately manifests itself as metabolic acidosis and hypotension. In addition to the above, some pathogens produce toxins that directly depress cardiac contractility, further compromising CO.

Blood pressure and the brain
In healthy adults and children cerebral blood flow is controlled by autoregulation. This means that cerebral blood flow is maintained within normal limits even in the face of systemic hyper- or hypotension. This control system operates less well in ill infants – especially those who are preterm. Rapid fluctuations in blood pressure (especially in the presence of hypoxia or acidosis) increase the risk of altered cerebral perfusion causing hypoxic injury or intraventricular haemorrhage (IVH) in preterm infants.

Circulatory changes at birth
In utero blood is oxygenated via the placenta. The foramen ovale and ductus arteriosus are patent and the lungs have a high resistance, so there is very little pulmonary blood flow. Blood bypasses the lungs by flowing straight from the right to left atrium via the foramen ovale, or by via the pulmonary artery into the aorta through the ductus arteriosus. At birth, as the infant aerates the lungs, the pulmonary vascular resistance falls and allows blood to flow through the lungs.

Flow via the foramen ovale gradually reduces and usually ceases. The ductus arteriosus contracts in response to increased oxygen levels in the blood. The pres-

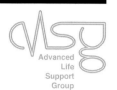

sure in the pulmonary artery also decreases and therefore flow through the duct diminishes. It is usually functionally closed within the first day of life. Failure to aerate the lungs at birth and to establish adequate blood flow through them results in hypoxia. If this is prolonged, the pulmonary circulation maintains a high resistance that manifests as persistent pulmonary hypertension. Congenital structural abnormalities can interfere with cardiovascular adaptation at birth (see Chapter 12).

Primary assessment circulation in children
- Look:
  - colour: cyanosis, pallor
  - plethora
  - dysmorphic features that may suggest congenital heart disease.
- Listen:
  - heart sounds, rate and rhythm
  - gallop
  - murmurs
  - measure blood pressure
- Feel:
  - capillary refill time
  - heart rate: note trends
  - pulse character: limb pulses – especially femoral
  - peripheral perfusion (cool extremities)
  - thrills
  - liver size.

Assessment of absolute values and trends in heart rate, colour, capillary refill time and peripheral perfusion will help diagnose impending shock (Table 11.3). BP is likely to be satisfactory if the mean BP is greater than gestation in the newborn. Review arterial or capillary blood gases: if the base excess (BE) > 5 mmol/l or the lactate > 2 mmol/l, this may indicate poor tissue perfusion.

Table 11.3 Healthy preterm infants on day 1 of life

Gestation (weeks)	n	Systolic range (mmHg)	Diastolic range (mmHg)	Heart rate (min–max)	Mean BP
<24	11	48–63	24–39	120–190	24
24–28	55	48–58	22–36	120–190	24–28
29–32	110	47–59	27–34	120–170	30
>32	68	48–60	24–34	120–170	30

Printed with kind permission from Paediatric and Neonatal Critical Care Transport, BMJ Books 2003.

Immediate management
- Vascular access: adequate, secure, vascular access is fundamental to safe transfer. Consider a central line or an umbilical venous catheter in newborn infants (possibly dual lumen).
- Arterial access should be placed wherever possible to allow sampling and invasive blood pressure monitoring.
- Stabilisation of the circulation:
  - consider volume infusion and inotrope support early.
  - consider transfusion if haemoglobin < 120 g/l in neonates or <80 g/l otherwise.

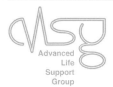

D – Disability
Primary survey

This involves the assessment and immediate management of a potentially compromised central nervous system (CNS). Peri- and antenatal history may raise the index of suspicion of CNS injury and guide ongoing assessment and treatment.

- Look:
  - posture
  - activity
  - abnormal movements (in infants excess sucking/chewing/staring/cycling of legs or arms/apnoea) or obvious seizures in all groups
  - pupillary abnormalities
  - blood gas result
- Listen:
  - verbalisation – tone of cry
- Feel:
  - fontanelle (in infants)
  - tone.

> DO NOT FORGET TO MEASURE THE CHILD'S PLASMA GLUCOSE.

Stabilisation of the nervous system

Attention to stabilisation of the airway, breathing and circulation should have corrected hypoxia and hypotension. Treat hypoglycaemia as a matter of urgency and also consider treating any other metabolic abnormalities, for example, hypocalcaemia or hypomagnesaemia. Treat significant seizures with anticonvulsants (after correcting hypoglycaemia). PCO_2 should be maintained in the normal range. A low PCO_2 may cause cerebral vasoconstriction and reduce brain oxygenation. A high PCO_2 causes cerebral vasodilatation and may increase intracranial pressure in traumatic head injuries.

Therapeutic hypothermia is currently practised in some centres in newborn infants, because it is thought to be neuroprotective in some asphyxiated children. Some centres now cool some infants after asphyxial injury to core temperatures of 33.5 ± 0.5°C. Outside specialist centres, this is not currently routine practice; however, close attention should be paid to avoiding hyperthermia because this is known to be damaging to the hypoxic infant brain. It is advisable to keep core temperature 36.5–37°C in these circumstances. The evidence to support this practice in older children after traumatic brain injury remains inconclusive.

E – Exposure

Conventionally this refers to a full inspection of the exposed body of an adult patient. This is also appropriate in children after traumatic injury. However, in the neonatal period exposure carries a different emphasis and should be considered in parallel to ABC. Very immature and low-birthweight babies are particularly vulnerable to cold. Hypothermia increases oxygen demand and adversely affects blood clotting. Low temperatures in preterm infants are associated with a poorer outcome, so minimisation of heat loss is an urgent priority in all infants and especially preterm infants. Preterm and low-birthweight infants have a high surface area and lose heat through the following mechanisms:

- Convection: from exposed skin to surrounding air. This is exacerbated in a draught.

- Radiation: from the surface of the baby via infrared waves to cooler surfaces. This is reversed by using a radiant heater.
- Evaporation: heat is lost as water evaporates from the skin – preterm infants are especially vulnerable to water loss. This may be minimised by the use of humidity or 'waterproofing' the infant with a plastic sheet or bubble wrap.
- Conduction: to cooler surfaces in direct contact with infant's skin. This is reduced using warm bedclothes and maintaining that temperature with a chemically activated gel mattress such as a Transwarmer.

The following are other practical measures to minimise thermal stress that should be considered:
- Minimise exposure time for examinations: use portholes if the infant is in an incubator
- Minimise draughts and warm room/ambulance
- Nurse in warmed humidified incubator
- Use a hat
- Prewarm transport incubator to 39–40°C
- Humidify incubator if possible
- Humidify inspired gases
- Use a radiant heat source if not in an incubator
- Continually monitor temperature
- Do not transfer a patient until the temperature is normal.

At delivery many centres now place very preterm infants into plastic bags without drying them; when the infant is then placed under a radiant heat source this creates a warm moist microenvironment for the infant which is very effective at maintaining temperature.

SECONDARY SURVEY

A thorough head-to-toe, front-to-back examination of the child should be carried out. After this, additional appropriate investigations should be undertaken or planned as part of the formulation of a definitive plan for continuing care. It is important to note that the child must be monitored to assess the effect of treatment and detect any deterioration. If this occurs re-evaluation of the primary survey is mandatory. By the end of the secondary survey you should have a working diagnosis plus a list of additional investigations and treatment. This will usually include the assessment of the most appropriate place for the infant to receive further care.

Box 11.4 Need for transfer

- Specialist treatment
- Specialist investigations
- More appropriate location for the delivery of level 0, 1, 2 or 3 care

---

SUMMARY

When assessing a child, it is vital rapidly to assess the situation using a structured ABCDE approach. This is best divided into two key phases:
- Primary survey: to identify and immediately treat life-threatening problems.
- Secondary survey and emergency treatment: to gain corroborative evidence for the primary diagnosis, identify new features and plan further care.

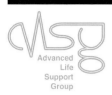

CHAPTER 12

Specific clinical conditions

> **LEARNING OBJECTIVES**
>
> In this chapter you will learn about clinical management of common paediatric and neonatal conditions.

The discussions in this chapter provide an overview of the background and clinical considerations of a number of important paediatric and neonatal conditions that may require transfer. This chapter is not intended to be exhaustive; rather it presents a subset of conditions that are included either because of their frequency or because they require specific management to achieve the best outcome.

In all cases the standard resuscitation algorithm of ABCDE should be followed. The information here supplements this approach and consequently assumes that the approach has already been appropriately applied.

BRONCHIOLITIS

This common seasonal illness is a major contributor to the increase in clinical activity during the winter months. Severely affected children often need to be cared for in a high dependency unit (HDU) or paediatric intensive care unit (PICU). Most cases occur between October and March, and around half are caused by the respiratory syncytial virus (RSV), with the remainder caused by other common respiratory viruses. The underlying pathophysiology is of bronchiolar obstruction secondary to inflammatory debris and oedema. Areas of atelectasis form, and ball-valve-type obstruction may lead to areas of hyperinflation.

Requirement for transfer to PICU for invasive ventilation is the result of either progressive respiratory failure with respiratory acidosis or, in younger infants, recurrent apnoea. Apnoeas may often be the presenting feature of the illness in young infants, occurring before there is any obvious respiratory distress. The need for ventilation can sometimes be avoided by using continuous positive airway pressure (CPAP) to reduce the work of breathing and prevent atelectasis. This may be delivered in HDUs in some centres, but in others will require transfer to a PICU. The children who are most likely to require intubation and ventilation

Paediatric and Neonatal Safe Transfer and Retrieval: The Practical Approach, Edited by Steve Byrne, Steve Fisher, Peter-Marc Fortune, Cassie Lawn and Sue Wieteska. © 2008 Blackwell Publishing, ISBN: 978-1-4051-6919-6.

are those with a history of chronic lung disease of prematurity (CLDP), newborn infants or infants with an underlying cardiorespiratory abnormality.

Once ventilated, oxygen saturations of 88–92% and permissive hypercapnia keeping pH > 7.2–7.25 are acceptable. Use of positive end-expiratory pressure (PEEP) in the range 6–15 cmH$_2$O often improves oxygenation and ventilation/perfusion ($\dot{V}/\dot{Q}$) mismatch by minimising atelectasis. A respiratory rate of 30 with an inspiratory time of 0.8 second is a reasonable starting point for ventilation. During transfer, ET tube obstruction by secretions should be anticipated. Regular ET suction using 0.9% saline is advisable. End-tidal CO$_2$ (ETCO$_2$) monitoring will often provide an early clue that suction is necessary. Transferring staff must ensure that there is a plentiful supply of appropriate gauge suction catheters, and portable suction must be available at all times. The best way to manage these children on PICUs is to allow spontaneous synchronised ventilation; however, during transfer they will usually be paralysed to prevent excessive movement and coughing, which may displace the ET tube.

A common issue encountered in these infants is whether to transfer using CPAP or escalate to invasive ventilation. The best place to deliver care will be determined by local circumstances. Non-invasive ventilation can be performed on general paediatric wards where provision has been made to permit high dependency care. The risk of transferring children with CPAP is that they become unstable en route and require ventilation as an emergency. The need to intubate and start ventilation in the back of an ambulance is best avoided! When children are started on CPAP in a referring centre with the resources to provide appropriate HDU care, it is appropriate to wait and see if they stabilise. Any significant deterioration should generate a prompt clinical review followed by intubation, ventilation and transfer where required. Transfer on CPAP under the direction of a consultant may be appropriate.

EPIGLOTTITIS

Although this has become much less common since the introduction of the *Haemophilus influenzae* type b (Hib) immunisation, it does still occur, and can be caused by other organisms. It has become more common in recent years secondary to Hib vaccine failures. The child typically presents with a very short history of fever, drooling and stridor. The child appears very flushed and hot. Upset to the child must be minimised, so painful or potentially upsetting examinations or procedures are absolutely contraindicated. Senior help should be summoned promptly. If there are signs of upper airway obstruction, the child should be intubated, by a consultant intensivist or anaesthetist, after gaseous induction.

It is recommended that an ENT (ear, nose and throat) surgeon also be present and ready to perform an emergency tracheostomy if necessary. Where possible, a nasotracheal tube, placed once the operator has secured the airway via an oral ET tube, will assist later management of the child on a PICU. Elective reintubation should not be undertaken if there is any doubt of success. The challenges here lie with the initial induction and intubation, and less with the transport – except to say that security of the ET tube is of paramount importance. The child should be sedated and paralysed for the transfer and the ET tube fixed with tape firmly to the face, ensuring that it does not move. ETCO$_2$ monitoring is mandatory to allow immediate recognition of a displaced or blocked tube. If accidental extubation were to occur, then a gum elastic bougie should be available to assist in correct replacement. If it is not possible either to reintubate or to ventilate by bag–valve–mask, a laryngeal mask may allow some ventilation to be achieved,

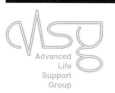

although, in the context of a severe epiglottitis, the only way to provide oxygenation may be via a needle cricothyroidotomy.

In practice, with an experienced retrieval team, the incidence of accidental extubation is extremely low. The likeliest points at which it might occur are when moving the child between bed and stretcher, and on loading and unloading the stretcher in the ambulance. At these times, one team member should be allocated the specific role of ensuring that all ventilator tubing and monitoring cables are in a secure position and not likely to snag. In moving the child from a bed to a trolley, it is advisable to disconnect the ventilator from the tube for the short time that it takes to move the child.

These children are septic, so, in addition to airway management, remember that they may require cardiovascular support. This may include fluid boluses and inotrope infusions. Consideration should be given to placing a central line before transfer.

UPPER AIRWAY DISEASE

Croup is the most common upper airway emergency requiring intubation and ventilation. Fortunately this is needed in only a small fraction of cases. The child typically presents with coryzal symptoms, low-grade fever, harsh barking cough and stridor.

The key indication for intubation is respiratory distress, which may characteristically manifest as severe sternal and intercostal recession plus or minus hypoxia. Eventually, even in a moderately severe case, the child may become exhausted and require intubation to maintain adequate ventilation. Airway obstruction is always worst when the child is upset and consequently trying to generate high gas flows through an obstructed upper airway. Temporary relief may be achieved through the use of nebulised adrenaline (epinephrine) (0.5 ml/kg of 1 : 1000 adrenaline up to maximum of 5 ml).

Many children with croup will be free of stridor for a period after this treatment. Some then develop worsening stridor after an initial response to adrenaline, probably not because of rebound hyperaemia of their upper airway mucosa, but because of severe underlying inflammation. The need for an adrenaline nebuliser should always prompt an immediate consultant review. The need for multiple adrenaline nebulisers almost invariably indicates the need for prompt intubation and ventilation.

With croup, as with all causes of upper airway obstruction, a requirement for supplementary oxygen in order to maintain normal saturations is worrying – all such children should be reviewed immediately by a consultant.

The glottic swelling often means that only a relatively narrow tube can be passed. Standard tubes are often too short for the child. Specially designed 'croup tubes' are available that are long tubes of narrow diameter.

The need for tube security applies here, as it does in epiglottitis and all other upper airway obstruction.

ACUTE-ON-CHRONIC RESPIRATORY FAILURE

Many admissions to the PICU result from respiratory infections in children who have pre-existing lung disease, most commonly CLDP. This is usually evident from the history given by the parents, although there may be additional clues from the appearance of the chest radiograph and the presence of a partially compensated respiratory acidosis.

Children with chronic lung disease often have coexistent areas of hyperinflation and collapse. The chest radiographs may be difficult to interpret. Careful inspection for a pneumothorax is important before departure. Consideration should be given to draining even a small pneumothorax in these circumstances. The chest radiograph should be used together with oxygen saturations and blood gas analysis to select appropriate ventilator settings. These infants may often respond well to a moderately high PEEP and relatively long inspiratory times; this will maintain a high mean airway pressure while allowing peak pressures to be kept to a minimum. As with children with bronchiolitis, aim for oxygen saturations of 88–92% and a strategy of permissive hypercapnia are a reasonable approach. Careful attention to appropriate sedation is especially important in children with chronic lung disease because they may have secondary pulmonary hypertension.

Many of these children will require a long period of stabilisation before transport. There is often a degree of experimentation needed with ventilator settings – no general 'ventilator recipe' suits all.

SEVERE PNEUMONIA

It is relatively unusual for a bacterial or viral pneumonia to cause respiratory failure severe enough to require ventilation in a previously well child beyond early infancy. Such a requirement should prompt enquiry into evidence of a pre-existing respiratory, neurological or immunological problem.

With a severe bacterial pneumonia, marked respiratory deterioration may be caused by an empyema. An ultrasound scan of the chest will allow evaluation of the presence and location of any pleural fluid. A chest drain to relieve even a small collection may produce a rapid, significant improvement.

Children with a bacterial pneumonia may have significant systemic sepsis, so their haemodynamic status must be evaluated carefully (heart rate, perfusion, urine output and lactate). Appropriate volume resuscitation should be administered and consideration given to the insertion of a central venous line and inotrope infusion.

ACUTE RESPIRATORY DISTRESS SYNDROME

Acute respiratory distress syndrome (ARDS) is the term used to describe severe respiratory failure associated with bilateral pulmonary infiltrates on chest radiograph, with no evidence of cardiogenic pulmonary oedema. It may result from extrapulmonary or pulmonary causes:
• Pulmonary:
  – pneumonia
  – aspiration of gastric contents
  – smoke inhalation
  – near drowning
• Extrapulmonary:
  – sepsis
  – trauma
  – burns.
The list of causes is far from exhaustive, but covers the most common seen in PICUs.

The pathophysiology is of a severe inflammatory oedema caused by vascular endothelial injury and increased capillary permeability. Ventilation–perfusion

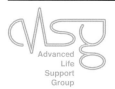

mismatch causes severe hypoxia and areas of consolidation develop in a dependent fashion, causing a heterogeneous decrease in pulmonary compliance. In extrapulmonary ARDS the treatment will be complicated by the predisposing cause, and the mortality of the condition is related to this rather than the presence of ARDS as such. The prognosis for pulmonary ARDS in a previously well child is very good if treated in a PICU.

When managing the respiratory system it is important to bear in mind the underlying pathophysiology. Simplistically, the lungs can be imagined as having three areas: fluid-filled consolidated lung in which the alveolar units are effectively unrecruitable; relatively well-inflated areas that are easily ventilated; and intermediate areas where increasing and maintaining airway pressure may permit recruitment of more alveolar units for gas exchange. These are heterogeneously distributed, but in a roughly gravity dependent manner – that is, the fluid-engorged consolidated areas are located in dependent areas and the well-inflated areas are in the uppermost regions (anteriorly in a supine child).

The decreased pulmonary compliance has led to the concept of setting ventilator pressures around the inflection point of the dynamic compliance curve (Figure 12.1).

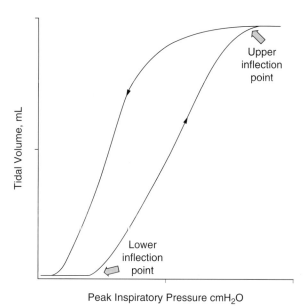

Fig. 12.1 Compliance diagram.

The aim is to ventilate the lungs as effectively as possible by recruiting as much of the intermediate area without causing overdistension of the easily ventilated units. Attempts to ventilate the 'unrecruitable' areas (by using high delivered tidal volumes) will result in overdistension of easily ventilated areas and will be counterproductive. There is now a significant body of laboratory and clinical evidence to show that trying to ventilate with 'normal' tidal volumes results in poorer outcome.

In practice this means setting PEEP levels high (10–15 cmH$_2$O) and tidal volumes low at 3–6 ml/kg, accepting oxygen saturations of 88–92% and allowing permissive hypercapnia. Surprisingly high pressures may often be needed to achieve these goals. Avoidance of disconnection of the ventilator circuit helps to maintain alveolar recruitment. Many of these children will be treated with high-frequency oscillatory ventilation (HFOV) once they arrive on a PICU. Transport ventilators that allow so-called active PEEP (pressure maintained by high continuous gas flow rather than an occlusive valve) may help achieve improved CO$_2$ clearance, but their gas consumption rates are high, so it must be ensured that there is enough oxygen for the trip.

The high intrathoracic pressures generated by ventilation in these children mean that they will often require increased intravascular filling pressures to maintain an adequate cardiac output.

CONGENITAL HEART DISEASE

Advances in paediatric cardiac surgery and postoperative care of these children have led some to argue that the time of greatest danger for these children is not perioperatively, but during the time period before they reach the specialist centre. Early discharge of babies who appear initially well means that many will present in extremis to Emergency Departments. One in four of babies dying in the first week of life from cardiac disease had not had their diagnosis recognised before presentation in extremis.

A provisional diagnosis may be available locally, but this is rarely made by a paediatric cardiologist, so management decisions may not be clear cut and should be discussed with a paediatric intensivist or cardiologist.

The detail of the underlying anatomy is unimportant in the initial stages of resuscitation and management – the principles of ABC are just the same as in other settings, with the qualification that normal oxygen saturations may not be achievable (or desirable).

The key feature in addition to ABC is that of ductal patency. Congenital heart disease presents acutely with any of the following:

- Cyanosis, but otherwise looks well (alert, active, minimal or no tachypnoea)
- Cyanosis and sick (respiratory distress)
- Shock.

In nearly all cases, maintenance of the patency of the ductus arteriosus that connects the systemic and pulmonary circulations is paramount. It is often the physiological closure of the ductus that precipitates clinical deterioration and presentation of the illness. Measures to reopen a closing ductus may therefore produce a rapid improvement in the child's condition.

Ductal patency is maintained by prostaglandin E_1 (alprostadil) 50–100 ng/kg/min or prostaglandin E_2 (dinoprostone) 5–50 ng/kg/min. The key side effects of these agents are apnoea and hypotension, which occur with increasing frequency as the dose increases. If apnoeas occur, intubation and ventilation should be performed, and hypotension should be treated by volume resuscitation and inotropes; the infusion must not be discontinued.

Cyanosed and well

An example of this is transposition of the great arteries. The infant who is cyanosed and well can be managed with a prostaglandin infusion, and observed for apnoeas, but does not necessarily need to be electively intubated. If the infant is stable for several hours on low or standard doses of prostaglandin, he or she can be transferred without intubation – apnoeas usually occur early after institution of high-dose prostaglandin.

Respiratory distress and cyanosis

Examples include pulmonary atresia, severe tetralogy of Fallot, and non-cardiac, for example, persistent pulmonary hypertension of the newborn. Infants with respiratory distress and cyanosis may have a pulmonary rather than a cardiac problem. A nitrogen washout test (breathing 100% oxygen for 10 min) that

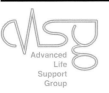

shows a rise in saturations and a $PaO_2 > 15\,kPa$ makes a respiratory cause more likely. However, failure to improve oxygenation may simply reflect an intrapulmonary shunt, or cardiac shunting secondary to pulmonary hypertension. It does not confirm cardiac disease. It is reasonable to start a prostaglandin infusion, intubate and ventilate the child for respiratory failure, and transfer to a specialist centre for a definitive diagnosis.

Shocked infants

Infants who present with shock may have sepsis or a duct-dependent circulation secondary to systemic outflow obstruction (for example, hypoplastic left heart syndrome, critical aortic stenosis, coarctation of the aorta). The hallmark signs are poor systemic perfusion, metabolic acidosis and weak or impalpable pulses. It is usually reasonable to start a prostaglandin infusion and to treat for sepsis with broad-spectrum antibiotics – there will often be a good response to prostaglandin in those with congenital heart disease and those with sepsis will often show some response to fluid boluses. However, distinguishing the two is only really possible with echocardiography.

Once some stability has been achieved by re-opening the duct and ensuring its patency, the focus shifts to balancing the systemic and pulmonary circulations. In hypoplastic left heart syndrome, two parallel circuits are in operation. Blood in the right ventricle can be pumped into the lungs via the pulmonary artery, or into the aorta via the ductus. Ideally this should be in a 1 : 1 ratio. Too much blood to the lungs will be at the expense of the systemic circulation, manifest by a continuing metabolic acidosis, poor urine output and relatively high oxygen saturations. Increasing the FiO_2 to try to achieve high saturations may lower pulmonary vascular resistance, and promote this systemic steal, so it is important to use a ventilator that allows low FiO_2 (or air) to be administered. Saturations of 70–80% are a reasonable target – bear in mind that this will be the saturation target that surgeons will be aiming for in the first stage of repair, and will sustain the child for several months or even years.

CARDIOMYOPATHY, MYOCARDITIS, PERICARDITIS

Intrinsic heart disease is rare in children compared with adults. Dilated cardiomyopathy and myocarditis may present as congestive cardiac failure at any age, and the clinical features overlap, making it difficult to differentiate the two at acute presentation. Other children will have had the diagnosis of dilated cardiomyopathy established long before they present to a PICU team. In both cases the challenge is to maintain sufficient cardiac output to maintain systemic oxygen delivery. ICU management will be along the same lines until there is improvement in the underlying condition, but some may eventually require full support with ECMO.

These diagnoses should be considered in a child with shock or pulmonary oedema, an enlarged liver (before any fluid resuscitation) and an enlarged cardiac contour on chest radiograph. Echocardiography and an ECG will confirm the diagnosis, and allow the estimation of cardiac contraction. This is quoted as fractional shortening (FS) in children (adults often have the ejection fraction reported). Fractional shortening is normally in the range 28–42% – it is simply a two-dimensional measure of how much the left ventricle contracts during systole as a fraction of its original dimensions.

Intubation and ventilation may be beneficial in children with a very low FS. This is achieved by reducing left ventricular afterload and also the work of breathing, which may be significant because of their pulmonary oedema. However, these benefits may be outweighed by the risk of induction and intubation – the vasodilatory and negative inotropic effects of the anaesthetic agents can cause cardiac arrest. Induction agents tend to be chosen to minimise these effects – fentanyl and ketamine tend to be popular in this situation. Resuscitation drugs should be drawn up in readiness, and the child transferred to the safest environment available.

Once ventilated, inotropes are started if they have not already been introduced. The choice of inotrope is determined by personal preference rather than evidence, but dopamine is a reasonable starting point in a dose of 5–10 mcg/kg/min. Adrenaline should be considered if there is no response. A starting dose of 0.1 mcg/kg per min should be employed and titrated up or down as needed. The desired therapeutic end-point is to achieve an adequate cardiac output. If available, this can be measured directly by the PiCCO or CardioQ systems. Otherwise, optimisation of cardiac output may be estimated through measurement of surrogate markers, such as heart rate, peripheral perfusion, arterial lactate concentration, urine output and blood pressure (continuously measured from an arterial line). Preload should be optimised judiciously using small (5 ml/kg) boluses of fluid and close monitoring of response of end-points. Ventilation often requires a high PEEP if there is pulmonary oedema. In children with severe bloody pulmonary oedema, constant suctioning of the ET tube is seldom helpful – the ventilator should be reconnected and high PEEP (10–15 cmH$_2$O) applied.

Children with pericarditis uncommonly present to intensive care; when they do it is because of a pericardial effusion causing tamponade. The most common setting for this is the cardiac ICU postoperatively, but occasionally effusions present weeks later in postoperative cardiac children. Other causes are connective tissue disorders and malignant invasion of the pericardium. As with children with cardiomyopathy, induction of anaesthesia to facilitate drainage can be a high-risk procedure, and unless in extremis it is probably advisable not to undertake this outside a specialist centre. The decision about whether to intubate these children before transfer will be dictated by their clinical status. Unless they are in extremis, it may be safer to transfer them, unintubated, as soon as possible to the specialist centre.

DYSRHYTHMIA

Dysrhythmia requiring PICU transfer is usually as a result of a severe supraventricular tachycardia (SVT) in infancy or ventricular tachycardia (VT) in children who have been poisoned by agents such as tricyclic antidepressants or who have an underlying cardiomyopathy or myocarditis.

SVT

This presents with a heart rate of 220–250/min in infants. They usually tolerate this poorly. It generally takes a few hours for them to develop marked cardiac failure. The APLS (Advanced Paediatric Life Support) SVT algorithm should be followed (Figure 12.2).

There can be a problem differentiating SVT from sinus tachycardia in children. Sinus tachycardia secondary to hypovolaemia or sepsis will typically vary in rate in response to fluid boluses or handling, whereas the rate in SVT remains fixed. It may be helpful to fax the ECG to a paediatric cardiologist. It is important to try to capture a rhythm strip for this purpose.

VT

VT should be treated according to the APLS algorithm (Figure 12.3).

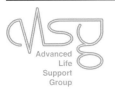

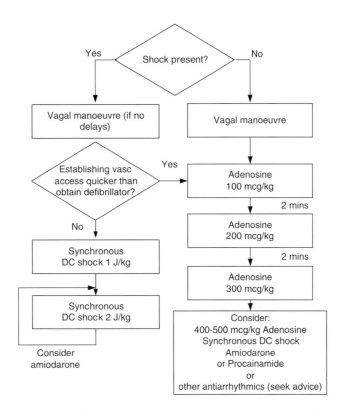

Fig. 12.2 Supraventricular tachycardia (SVT) algorithm.

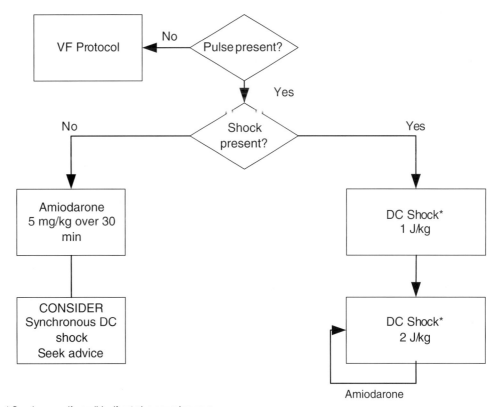

* Synchronous if possible, if not give asynchronous

Fig. 12.3 Ventricular tachycardia (VT) algorithm.

SPECIFIC NEONATAL CLINICAL CONDITIONS

Airway and breathing in the neonatal period

In the neonatal period it is vital to appreciate the immaturity of the lungs and the fact that they are easily damaged (particularly in the extreme preterm infant). Ventilatory strategies are therefore aimed at minimising pulmonary trauma (volutrauma) while ensuring adequate oxygenation and ventilation. A strategy of permissive hypercapnia and relative hypoxia is employed in the preterm infant.

Those involved in transport may not have been involved with the initial resuscitation and stabilisation following delivery. The babies who need to be moved will already be receiving a variable degree of airway support. The transport team must assess the adequacy of pre-existing support and augment it as necessary, to optimise the baby's status and minimise risk.

The clinical signs of respiratory inadequacy are similar to those of other children. Narrow compliant airways and secretions may compromise breathing. The very compliant chest wall results in rapid, inefficient breaths with accompanying grunting and recession. Fatigue may be reflected by respiratory pauses or apnoeas. There may be a compensatory tachycardia, with poor perfusion and visible cyanosis.

Measured parameters may help assessment, in particular of blood gases, oxygen saturation and (where measured) transcutaneous CO_2 ($TcCO_2$) and O_2 (TcO_2). Trends are often more important than individual readings. Table 12.1 gives the normal/target values.

Table 12.1 Normal/target values for preterm and term infants

Parameter	Preterm	Term
Target temperature (°C)	36–37	36–37
Target SaO_2 (%)	85–93	>95 (non-cardiac)
Target PaO_2 (kPa)[a]	6–8 (45–60)	8–12 (60–90)
Target $PaCO_2$ (kPa)[a]	4.6–8 (35–60) if compensated	4.6–6.0 (35–45)
Target blood sugar (mmol/l)	>2.6	>2.6

[a]Values in parentheses are mmHg.

Strategies that may be used during transport

- Prone nursing: improves mechanical efficiency
- Ambient oxygen supplementation into an incubator
- Oxygen supplementation via nasal prongs
- CPAP airway support
- Mechanical ventilation.

General advice

Where there are concerns about the stability of the airway, definitive support should be provided by an ET tube. Intubation is better done before transfer rather than as an emergency. The tube should be of appropriate diameter (Table 12.2) and length. Length at the lips (in centimetres) for oral tracheal tubes may be

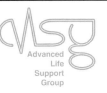

Table 12.2 Guide to endotracheal tube internal diameter by weight

Tube diameter (mm)	Weight of baby (g)
2.5	<1500
3.0	1500–2499
3.5	>2500

estimated as (6 + weight in kilograms) cm, except in extreme preterm babies – see Appendix 3). Correct positioning should always be confirmed by chest radiograph (tip of the ET tube midway between the carina and the level of the medial end of the clavicles).

Very preterm neonates and all babies with unstable airways, apnoeic episodes, rising inspired oxygen requirements or increasing $PaCO_2$ should usually be electively intubated and ventilated, even if only for the duration of the move. Any deviation from this course of action must be discussed and agreed with the consultant supervising the transfer.

Circulatory support in the neonatal period

Fortunately, with neonates it is relatively infrequent that the circulation needs support. They are not usually volume depleted, although in septic conditions third space losses, and reduced vascular tone, can manifest as significant intravascular volume depletion. A bolus of 10 ml/kg of fluid may optimise cardiac output.

The ability of the circulation to deliver oxygen is critical. Anaemia reduces the oxygen-carrying capacity of the blood. Normal newborn haemoglobins run around 150–160 g/l with the haematocrit around 50–60%. A significantly low plasma haemoglobin accompanied by a raised inspired oxygen requirement should prompt consideration of a packed cell transfusion: 15–25 ml/kg of packed cells is likely to increase the haemoglobin by around 40–60 g/l.

Once the circulating volume has been optimised, consider inotropic support. The same basic principles arise here as elsewhere. First-line drugs often used in the neonatal period include dopamine 5–10 mcg/kg per min and dobutamine 5–10 mcg/kg per min. The effects of these drugs are sometimes unpredictable so it is essential to titrate carefully and monitor heart rate, blood pressure (BP), urine output and other signs of perfusion. The aim is to improve cardiac output, not increase BP in isolation. As a rule of thumb the mean BP in millimetres of mercury should be greater than or equal to the gestational age in weeks on the first day of life. Low readings without a decrease in urine output and/or metabolic acidosis should probably not be treated.

Disease-specific strategies
Respiratory distress syndrome (hyaline membrane disease)

Also known as surfactant-deficient lung disease. Primary surfactant deficiency results in stiff lungs (with a low functional residual capacity), increased work of breathing, oxygen dependency and respiratory failure.

Extreme preterm infants should be intubated and ventilated and given exogenous surfactant. Larger and more mature infants may cope with CPAP support.

If transporting an unintubated infant, the transfer team must be competent to establish a definitive intubated airway.

When ventilating neonates the aim is to use minimal distending pressures in order to achieve adequate gas exchange without alveolar overexpansion. If necessary, especially on transport ventilators, which deliver intermittent mandatory ventilation (IMV) only, sedate (and if necessary paralyse) to avoid asynchrony. Commonly used drugs include morphine, diazepam, fentanyl, atracurium and vecuronium.

Typical ventilator strategies use inspiratory times of 0.3–0.35 s, rates of 40–60 breaths/min, a PEEP of 4–6 cmH$_2$O, and the lowest peak inspiratory pressure (PIP) that achieves acceptable blood gases.

Where appropriate, surfactant ($\geq$100 mg/kg) should be administered. This should be instilled before transfer to enable its effect on lung compliance to be assessed before the journey begins.

Cardiac function is usually well maintained. Monitoring should be via a peripheral arterial line or umbilical artery catheter (UAC). If there is evidence of poor perfusion (rising heart rate, increased toe/core temperature gap, skin pallor) a fluid bolus may be justified to optimise preload and enhance cardiac output. Early consideration should be given to inotropic support.

Maintenance fluids are usually given as 10% dextrose. In the first 24–48 hours it is not usually necessary to add sodium or potassium – a rate of 60–100 ml/kg per day depending on gestation. Maintenance of blood sugar is important (aim to keep above 2.6 mmol/l).

The possibility of infection should always be considered in these infants. It may be difficult to differentiate between congenital pneumonia and respiratory distress syndrome on chest radiograph, so most of these babies should be treated with antibiotics. A typical antibiotic regimen would be intravenous benzylpenicillin and gentamicin.

Pneumothorax

Pneumothoraces may complicate any respiratory illness, and are seen most commonly where the lungs are stiff. An active baby who is not maintaining respiratory synchrony with the ventilator is also at increased risk. They may also occur spontaneously.

Presentation may be precipitous with acute collapse, desaturation and evidence of air leak on chest examination. Deterioration in any baby with respiratory illness should raise the suspicion of a pneumothorax. In extreme cases cardiac tamponade may occur secondary to a tension pneumothorax. Clinical signs of a tension pneumothorax include asymmetry of chest wall movement and breath sounds, and ipsilateral increased transillumination. On occasions significant pneumothoraces are still sometimes not identified without a chest radiograph.

In a ventilated baby needing transfer, pneumothoraces will usually require drainage. If the baby has a tension pneumothorax a needle aspiration will be required to stabilise the situation before insertion of a definitive chest drain.

Meconium aspiration syndrome

Meconium is typically passed by term babies under stress. If hypoxic and gasping *in utero* aspiration may occur. Not all babies who may have aspirated meconium will develop the full-blown meconium aspiration syndrome (MAS), which causes a pneumonitis. There is a patchy effect with areas of collapse and air trapping. Both pulmonary and cardiac shunting will result in a ventilation–perfusion mismatch. Babies may be affected to a degree that requires ventilatory support. It is

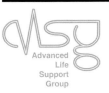

likely that the baby will have pulmonary hypertension; if not this may present later and can be very severe. Air trapping can be a problem with risk of air leak (pneumothorax and/or pneumomediastinum). The presence of MAS may indicate a primary hypoxic ischaemic insult that may also cause coexisting encephalopathy and other organ dysfunction (especially myocardial and renal).

If there is respiratory inadequacy, support is required. The primary problem is usually oxygenation and not CO_2 clearance. Air trapping can be very difficult to deal with. Stiff lungs require longer inspiratory times and higher pressure to oxygenate with concomitant risk of air leak. This must be achieved while allowing sufficient time for expiration, which may be abnormally long. Surfactant can help (many suggest a dose of up to 200 mg/kg), but the effect is sometimes unpredictable and more than two doses may be needed because it is inactivated rapidly by meconium. A high FiO_2 can be justified to minimise the risk of persistent pulmonary hypertension of the newborn (PPHN) and encourage pulmonary vasodilatation. This should be titrated to maintain a high normal PaO_2. The pH should be maintained at 7.35–7.45 by manipulation of CO_2. Sedation with morphine and paralysis with vecuronium or atracurium are vital to minimise pulmonary hypertension.

A significant number of these babies will require HFOV and possibly nitric oxide (NO) to stabilise their condition. Although the latter can be delivered en route, the former cannot and the baby will need to be stabilised on a conventional ventilator before transfer. There is strong evidence that babies with severe MAS benefit from management using ECMO and so these infants should be discussed with an ECMO centre early.

Cardiac function may be compromised because of the high ventilatory pressures that are required. The myocardium may also be damaged secondary to hypoxaemia. It is essential to ensure a good cardiac output. Ventilated infants should have arterial access and central venous access secured. Fluid boluses are likely to be required to increase cardiac preload and optimise cardiac output. Inotropic support is usually required in severe cases. These infants often have significant cerebral injury (hypoxic ischaemic encephalopathy) and must be watched for signs of seizures.

In mature infants it is customary to maintain fluids within the low/restricted range initially (40 ml/kg per day is a typical figure), but hypoglycaemia can be a problem and needs to be managed appropriately.

Persistent pulmonary hypertension of the newborn

After birth all infants have a degree of pulmonary hypertension. In some this can cause problems because the pulmonary pressures are so high that they cause a reversal of the normal physiological flow patterns and right–left shunting occurs at intracardiac (foramen ovale) or extracardiac (ductal) levels. Therapeutic strategies are aimed at reversing this. This condition is known variously as PPHN, persistent fetal circulation (PFC) and persistent transitional circulation (PTC). It can occur as an isolated phenomenon after perinatal stress, or associated with other problems such as sepsis, MAS or respiratory distress syndrome. Precipitating factors include metabolic acidosis, hypoxia and hypercapnia. Diagnosis should ideally be confirmed by echocardiography. The differential diagnosis of PPHN is that of anomalous pulmonary venous drainage; both result in an enlarged right atrium with reverse shunting but treatment strategies are different.

In general optimise respiratory and circulatory support and treat any primary conditions if possible. Ventilatory strategies should aim to maintain oxygenation at high levels to encourage pulmonary vasodilatation. Acidosis will precipitate pulmonary vasoconstriction, so the pH should be maintained at 7.35–7.45. This may be achieved through manipulation of CO_2.

Systemic blood pressure should be maintained with early use of inotropes. The use of selective pulmonary vasodilators may also be necessary. If available, NO should be used. Obviously if moving a baby who is already on NO, then the transport system must be capable of maintaining this.

If this is not available, the alternatives that may help include prostacyclin, adenosine or magnesium sulphate. These drugs also have systemic actions and their effect is therefore not predictable. These should be used only by personnel familiar with their actions.

Surgical problems

Congenital diaphragmatic hernia

It is increasingly unusual to have to move babies with this condition over a long distance after birth. Most are diagnosed antenatally and electively delivered in or very close to a specialist surgical centre. However, even within a surgical centre these infants may need moving between intensive care and theatre.

Problems arise as a result of pulmonary hypoplasia (especially on the side of the hernia), the presence of abdominal contents in the thoracic cavity and associated pulmonary hypertension. Intubation should be performed as soon as possible to permit lung inflation without gastric distension, which may occur with bag–valve–mask support. This is especially true as the lungs may have poor compliance and be quite stiff to bag. Such distension may further compromise breathing because of the effect of the distended gut compressing the lung tissue.

High ventilation pressures with long inspiratory times may be required. There is a significant risk of air leak in this situation. Pneumothoraces will require prompt drainage. Surfactant may be helpful in optimising alveolar recruitment. In the non-transport setting oscillatory ventilation may be used, but is currently unavailable for transport (although high-frequency jet ventilation is used in transport by some teams). If on HFOV, infants must be converted from this mode before any move and long enough before the move to assess stability. A nasogastric tube should be passed early to minimise gastric distension. It should be aspirated regularly and left on free drainage between times. Target values for gas exchange are to keep the PaO_2 in the high normal range, pH around 7.35–7.45 and $PaCO_2$ in the low–normal range to maintain the pH. This will maximise pulmonary vasodilatation and minimise any tendency to PPHN. Sedation and paralysis will be required in ventilated babies.

Full monitoring with arterial access is essential. Maintenance fluids should be provided with 10% dextrose. If there is evidence of pulmonary hypertension, appropriate strategies should be employed. Additional boluses of fluid, early inotropic support and NO may be required.

Babies with a congenital diaphragmatic hernia may have associated cardiac defects. Ideally an echocardiogram should be performed to assess the presence or absence of this before transfer.

Oesophageal atresia/tracheo-oesophageal fistulas

These are often identified antenatally (during investigation of polyhydramnios), but may also be diagnosed postnatally after cyanotic or aspiration episodes. With oesophageal atresia problems arise because the infant cannot swallow his or her own saliva, which then pools and may be aspirated. Where there is a coexisting fistula, respiratory difficulties may be compounded by gaseous distension of the stomach. This causes vagal overactivity, and splints the diaphragm, which can precipitate a cardiac arrest. It is impossible to aspirate the stomach and thus this

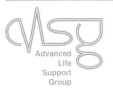

tendency must be minimised. Decompression and aspiration of any proximal pouch should be undertaken. A Replogle tube under continuous suction should be used (Figure 12.4). Where possible these infants should be allowed to breathe spontaneously. Positive pressure ventilation is less desirable, particularly where a fistula may cause gastric distension and splinting.

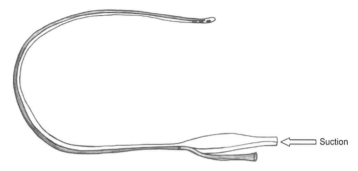

Fig. 12.4 Replogle tube.

Circulation is not usually a problem. There may be associated cardiac defects, which should ideally be identified/excluded before any move. Maintenance fluids should be administered intravenously at normal rates.

Exomphalos/Gastroschisis
Exomphalos (herniation of the abdominal contents into the umbilical cord) and gastroschisis (herniation of the abdominal contents through an abdominal wall defect beside the umbilical cord) require similar approaches. Gastroschisis requires a more urgent transfer to a surgical unit. However, it is important to note that exomphalos is more frequently associated with other congenital abnormalities. Both of these lesions are usually diagnosed on antenatal ultrasound examinations.

Airway and breathing are not usually a problem. Most infants do not require support unless there are other coexisting problems.

The circulation may require support. Fluid losses from the exposed abdominal contents may be significant (especially with a gastroschisis, where intestines are exposed). It is important to ensure that there is adequate venous access (preferably one central and one peripheral line). Maintenance fluids of 60–90 ml/kg per day of 10% dextrose should be given to maintain blood glucose. Boluses of fluid may be required to replace high insensible losses. It is good practice to review this requirement and increase maintenance fluid to cover these losses. An increasing metabolic acidosis or rising lactate must be investigated with diligence because it may indicate bowel ischaemia.

Treatment priorities are to protect the bowel from damage and minimise heat and fluid loss. The bowel may be wrapped in clingfilm to reduce evaporative and convective heat loss. The bowel should be positioned and covered to prevent it twisting on its pedicle, which could compromise the vascular supply. In a transport incubator, the infant may typically be nursed on their side. The clear material also allows a regular visual inspection of the bowel.

A nasogastric tube should be inserted and aspirated regularly because distension of the bowel could cause mechanical effects and tension on the vascular pedicle. Compromised bowel may appear dusky or even black and should prompt urgent action. It is wise to discuss the care of these babies with a paediatric surgeon, especially if bowel viability is in question.

Exomphalos may be associated with other conditions such as Beckwith–Weidemann syndrome. These hyperinsulinaemic infants are at high risk of hypoglycaemia, which must be identified and treated aggressively. Increased fluid volumes, higher concentrations of dextrose and occasionally glucagon may be required.

Gastrointestinal obstruction

Gastrointestinal obstruction may occur as part of a number of congenital conditions or as a consequence of other problems. Small and large bowel atresias, malrotation or meconium ileus may all present with a distended abdomen, failure to tolerate feeds, vomiting, discomfort, or more significant problems arising as a result of secondary compromise to the gut or of electrolyte disturbance.

In some cases bowel distension may splint the diaphragm and cause respiratory embarrassment. There are also risks of vomiting and aspiration. Stopping enteral intake is mandatory. Decompression via a nasogastric tube may reduce distension and will reduce the chance of aspiration.

If there has been significant vomiting or other fluid loss then the circulation may be compromised and resuscitation fluids may be required. Intravenous access is essential with adequate fluid to replace any deficit and to keep up with maintenance requirements and any continuing losses. If there have been/are significant nasogastric losses, there may be a resultant electrolyte disturbance. Sodium and potassium losses can be significant. Nasogastric aspirates should be replaced with 0.9% saline with added potassium.

Necrotising enterocolitis

Necrotising enterocolitis (NEC) is an insidious condition that shows a predilection for preterm babies. The abdomen distends, the baby stops tolerating enteral feeds and may have bilious vomiting or aspirates. If a radiograph is taken it may show pathognomonic features such as intramural gas or gas in the biliary tree. The bowel inflammation is associated with marked changes in bowel wall permeability and there may be marked fluid loss into the bowel.

Where the abdomen is significantly distended, ventilation may be required as a result of respiratory compromise. Relatively high pressures may be needed in response to the diaphragmatic splinting. A nasogastric tube should be passed and maintained on continuous drainage to minimise the intraluminal volume.

Treatment with resuscitation fluid may be required if fluid loss into the bowel has been significant. There may be thrombocytopenia and even disseminated intravascular coagulation in severe cases. There is an increased risk of infection secondary to bacterial translocation and it is recommended that these babies start antibiotics to cover particularly Gram-negative, Gram-positive and anaerobic organisms.

Many babies who are initially treated as possible NEC cases resolve rapidly with medical intervention. The presence of NEC may be uncertain in these cases. However, some babies do have definite disease and it is routine to keep these babies nil by mouth (and hence needing total parenteral nutrition) for 7–14 days. Such babies may need transfer to a surgical centre for insertion of a central line (usually semi-electively). In more serious cases a surgical referral is made for bowel perforation with or without evidence of peritonitis. Such babies may appear relatively well, or be in extremis, and can present significant challenges to the transfer team.

SUMMARY

In this chapter you have learnt about specific clinical conditions in relation to transfer.

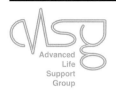

PART V
Special considerations

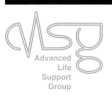

CHAPTER 13

Parent support

LEARNING OBJECTIVES

In this chapter you will learn about the importance of regular, clear communication with family members, throughout the transfer process.

INTRODUCTION

The transfer of a sick child can be a very difficult time for families and parents. It is not uncommon that the situation has progressed from that of having a normal healthy child, or expecting a healthy baby, to one of having a critically ill child receiving intensive care. Even if the condition is not life threatening, it may often appear so to the family. They will be stressed and frightened, and they may also be very tired. On occasions these factors may manifest as anger. It is vital that the clinical team recognise this and do not react and reflect anger back.

Communication should be clear, honest and open. Speculation and unrealistic assurances should be avoided. The need to transfer a critically sick child may not have been anticipated by the parents. The reasons for the transfer should be shared and explained. At the time of broaching the subject it is likely that the local team will continue caring for the child for some time, so great care is key to avoid undermining parental confidence in their local centre. It is also important because the child will most likely return to their care in the future. Wherever possible informed consent for the transfer should be sought, although this need not necessarily require the completion of a consent form (local trust policy should be followed in this regard).

Communication with families should usually be undertaken by the most senior member of the attending team, wherever possible. Honesty is vital throughout the process; the risks and benefits of transfer should be openly discussed.

COMMUNICATIONS BY THE TRANSFER TEAM

Before transfer

On arrival the transfer team should introduce themselves to the child's parents. Detailed discussions are usually best deferred until after the team have had an opportunity to assess the child clinically. Giving the parents some indication of

---

Paediatric and Neonatal Safe Transfer and Retrieval: The Practical Approach, Edited by Steve Byrne, Steve Fisher, Peter-Marc Fortune, Cassie Lawn and Sue Wieteska. © 2008 Blackwell Publishing, ISBN: 978-1-4051-6919-6.

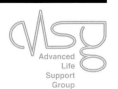

the timing of such discussions can be helpful. Do not underestimate the work that you have to do in this regard.

Once you are fully appraised of the clinical situation, a more detailed discussion may be undertaken with the parents. It is vital that, before this discussion, you are aware of previous conversations that the parents have had with the local team and what they have understood. This might be facilitated best by asking the parents what they have already been told. Even the most informed of parents may erroneously process information at times of stress and anxiety, so their understanding may be at considerable variance to the content of the conversation as described by the local team. In very complex situations, just the sheer volume of information can be bewildering. Expectations from previous conversations may need to be carefully managed, especially in an evolving clinical setting. Furthermore, it is not uncommon for parents to feel that once a transfer team arrives 'everything is going to be fine'. Once again, any need to revise a prognosis downwards should be handled without inadvertent criticism of local care.

It is quite natural to want to reassure parents. Honesty is vital, so any reassurance must be done within the limits of a child's likely outcome. In grave situations inappropriate optimism may give false hope that will make later management very difficult. This is especially true where a withdrawal of advanced support becomes appropriate.

Most parents will wish to accompany their child on a transfer; there is no standard guidance as to whether or not they should, because whether it is possible depends on many factors. Local team policy will influence this, as will practical issues around space, the child's clinical status and the mode of transfer. Wherever possible parents should accompany a conscious child to minimise the child's distress. Space is at a premium on many transfers, which may make it impossible to take a parent in the transport vehicle.

The fact that a child has a significant risk of dying during the transfer should not prevent the parent accompanying him or her. In fact on these occasions there could be very powerful arguments to support their presence. The time taken to transfer the child may be a significant part of a child's remaining life and parents should be excluded only if it is absolutely necessary. Furthermore, should the child die en route the presence of the parent may make their acceptance and understanding of the situation easier.

Mothers of newborn infants should not accompany them on transfer unless the mother is medically fit to do so, or there is a midwife to care for the mother during transfer. The latter is rarely possible because there is insufficient space in the back of an ambulance for a mother, a midwife and adult resuscitation equipment as well as a neonatal transport incubator, equipment and team.

When a parent is transported with their child it is vital to discuss 'ground rules' before setting off. It must be made clear that, should a significant deterioration take place, the parent must allow the team unhindered access to the child and their equipment. In an aircraft they will usually be in a seat somewhat separated from their child and this will not be an issue. However, on road ambulance transfers they should be advised that they will be required to vacate the back of the ambulance to allow the team to work. Very careful consideration should be given to allowing agitated or aggressive parents to travel with the team.

Many transfer teams carry hospital information packs for their regional units, with contact numbers, maps and travel information. It is helpful if these can be given to parents before the child's departure to enable parents to plan their journey and rejoin their child if they are not going on the transfer, or to pass the

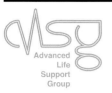

information on to other family members if they are. Clear information about how and when to reach their child at the receiving centre is helpful. Where possible transport should be arranged for the parents that does not involve their driving. If they do drive, gentle, non-patronising advice should be given about their driving style. They should be advised not to try to 'chase the ambulance' because this is both dangerous and illegal.

It is good practice to ensure that parents do not leave the referring hospital before the transport team. There have been a number of incidents where the child has deteriorated or even died before departure of the retrieval team, but after the family had left. The family then arrives at the receiving centre to be given the terrible information by an unfamiliar team, only to have to return to the referring hospital to be with their child.

During transfer

It is not always possible or appropriate to contact parents during a transfer; however, a brief update, even if only via text, is greatly appreciated by families. This is usually non-clinical information, for example, safe arrival. Detailed clinical information is best reserved for face-to-face communications.

Communication after transfer

Most teams will communicate with parents at the completion of a transfer, not only to say how the transfer went but also to give specific information about their child's exact location in the new facility as well as contact names and numbers of the new medical/nursing team.

RESPECTING PARENTAL WISHES

Parental wishes and expectations should always be treated with the utmost respect. If there appears to be a disparity between the clinical needs of the child, as perceived by the transfer team, and parental wishes this must always be promptly referred to the consultant in charge for urgent consideration and direction.

Cultural and religious views should also be considered when talking to parents. Where possible a qualified interpreter should be sought if English is not the parent's first language.

CONSENT

Most transfers of children take place with no more than verbal parental consent. On rare occasions parents may raise an objection to transfer, usually because they do not believe that it is in their child's best interests. This is most likely to arise because of a lack of understanding of the need for transfer. It will usually be resolved by further discussion and explanation of key issues.

It is possible that a parent may refuse to agree to the child being transferred even after lengthy discussions. In these circumstances, if a child is at risk of significant harm from not being transferred it may be acceptable to do so against parental wishes. The most senior member of the transfer team must be involved in the decision-making process and a clear written record must be kept of all discussions and reasons for the decisions made. Parents must be kept informed of any decision taken against their wishes and the reasons for those decisions. It is sometimes helpful in these circumstances to involve other family members or religious/pastoral leaders in these discussions.

Specific consent may be needed from parents for procedures that are planned at the receiving centre, for example, extracorporeal membrane oxygenation (ECMO) or surgery. If a parent is not accompanying a child on a transfer, this can be a problem. If the procedure cannot wait for a face-to-face meeting, usual practice would be for the clinician carrying out the procedure to obtain verbal consent over the telephone. It is helpful to warn parents that this may happen and to ensure that the transfer team have the relevant contact information.

Children aged over 16, or those younger than 16 who are deemed competent to understand the risks and benefits of a procedure, may give consent to their own treatment. However, children in acute transfer situations are usually too unwell to do so. Children without parents or those in state care can have consent given by a legal guardian or parent who holds parental responsibility. Both parents can give consent to treatment of their child if they are married. Unmarried fathers can give consent only if they are named on the child's birth certificate, have formally adopted the child or have been given parental responsibility by the Courts. This can be an issue in newborn infants before registration of the birth. Further information about consent issues can be found on the General Medical Council's website (www.gmc-uk.org).

ADVERSE OUTCOMES

If there has been open and honest discussion before and during the transfer a poor outcome should not come as a bolt from the blue. This will not reduce the impact of bad news but being poorly prepared may worsen distress. In the event of an unexpected adverse incident, the same principles of clear, open and honest communication, which should underpin the whole transfer process, still apply. If the child dies before the parents arrive, it will usually be better to wait for face-to-face contact rather than contacting them en route.

SUMMARY

In this chapter we have highlighted the importance of clear, open, honest communication with parents throughout the transfer process. This underpins the establishment of a good relationship with parents that may help to minimise distress at an extremely difficult time. Preparing children and their families with honest clinical information as well as practical information will help parents regain some control in what can be an extremely frightening situation.

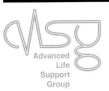

CHAPTER 14

Air transfers: an introduction

LEARNING OBJECTIVES

In this chapter you will learn:
- How to assess the benefits and disadvantages of air transfer
- The importance of the structured approach to aviation transfer medicine
- The safety aspects around helicopter landings

AIR TRANSFERS

Air transfers may be divided into two types based on the type of aircraft: fixed wing and rotary winged (helicopters). Within England and Wales, fixed-wing aircraft are not commonly used for domestic transfers; however, a number of patients are repatriated from overseas by this means. Paediatric air transfers are usually undertaken in order to shorten the time taken to perform the transport. This may be for reason of distance, road type or adverse traffic conditions. On occasions they may also be undertaken to travel to offshore sites.

Generally, air transport should be considered for longer journeys. Fixed-wing aircraft, preferably pressurised, should be considered for transfer distances greater than 150 miles (240 km). It is always important to remember that the perceived speed of air transfer must be balanced against organisational delays and intervehicle transfers at either end of the journey.

Helicopters

The use of helicopters for the transfer of patients has been the subject of some debate. The transfer of patients by helicopter has advantages in sparsely populated areas or a maritime environment. A helicopter can deliver medical, nursing or paramedical teams to enable roadside resuscitation to proceed. However, in an urban environment, helicopters may have no advantage over a well-equipped road-based service (see Appendix H). Most helicopters used for medical transfers in the UK have the following disadvantages:
- Access to the patient is limited
- They have a limited range without re-fuelling
- As there is limited availability of landing places, road transfers at the start and end of each flight are often needed

---

Paediatric and Neonatal Safe Transfer and Retrieval: The Practical Approach, Edited by Steve Byrne, Steve Fisher, Peter-Marc Fortune, Cassie Lawn and Sue Wieteska. © 2008 Blackwell Publishing, ISBN: 978-1-4051-6919-6.

- The possibility of any therapeutic interventions is extremely limited
- The vehicle cannot be halted during the transfer
- They have high running costs.

Road transport has the following advantages:
- Healthcare staff are more familiar with this environment
- Rapid mobilisation time
- Transfer is usually door to door
- Patient monitoring and observation are easier
- The vehicle can be halted to undertake therapeutic interventions
- Less disruption from adverse weather conditions
- Lower overall cost.

Civil air ambulances

In the UK, there are currently 18 civil air ambulance services, undertaking approximately 125 000 medical missions per year. Fifty per cent of all missions are related to road traffic accidents. Heart attack victims and 'collapsed' patients in remote areas also make up a significant proportion of the workload. Air ambulance helicopter services are classed as civil operations; they are usually charitably funded and organised by private organisations, which are in turn contracted by an NHS ambulance trust. Most of their work involves attending casualties in remote areas, although some interhospital transfers are also performed. The scope of work undertaken by air ambulances is limited by the following:
- Funding
- Availability of aircraft or pilots
- Range
- Weather – time of day
- Limited monitoring and ventilatory support.

In general, in England and Wales, civil charitable air ambulance operations are restricted to daylight hours because the aircraft have to find a landing site visually when they arrive at the scene. It is possible to operate from designated helipads after dark, provided that these are suitably lit either from the ground or from the helicopter. There is known to be a significant increase in helicopter accidents during night-time missions and in poor weather conditions.

Military provision

The Royal Air Force (RAF) maintains a year-round, 24-hour search and rescue service covering the whole of the UK and a large part of the surrounding sea. The service exists primarily to assist military and civilian aircrew who get into difficulty, although a large proportion of its work involves assisting shipping or people who find themselves in a wide variety of difficulties, both on land and at sea. The RAF and the Royal Naval Air Service (RNAS) Search and Rescue service 'assist' more than 1400 people each year, most of whom are transferred to hospital. In most rescues the RAF Aeronautical Rescue Centre (ARCC) at Kinloss in Scotland controls all aerial resources and works closely with the emergency services. RAF helicopters are operated by HM Forces under Ministry of Defence (MOD) regulations. In general terms, they are operated to standards that may permit them to fly into sites, and under weather conditions that would not be acceptable to civil operators.

Arranging a helicopter transfer

Air ambulance and helicopter emergency medical services (HEMS) may be available free to the NHS, through funding supported by charitable donations. Any

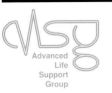

cost should be identified as early as possible along with an agreement to pay from the appropriate budget holder. Military 'assistance' is often free of charge; however, interfacility transfers are usually charged for. (Current fees are in the region of £3000 per flying hour.) The requesting hospital NHS trust will be expected to honour payment, so military transfers must be approved by the budget holder.

> All requests for helicopter transfer must be made to the local ambulance service trust by a senior member of staff who can authorise payment if required

APPLYING THE ACCEPT APPROACH TO AIR TRANSFERS

A – assess patient and situation

The job of the air crew is to provide facilities for transfer. They may have knowledge of advanced life support, but they should not be expected to provide expert medical or nursing care during transfer. The air ambulance service will usually arrange connecting transport with road ambulances if required. However, it is vital that this aspect of the transfer is discussed, agreed and documented to prevent unnecessary delays.

The following is the information likely to be needed when contacting air ambulance services:

- Name and age (DOB) of patient
- Location of patient and planned destination
- Diagnosis
- Condition severity
- Team details (location and number)
- Equipment accompanying patient (weight may be limited)
- Requests for family or carer to accompany
- Aggressive or infectious patients must be discussed with the pilot in command at the planning stage.

C – control of the situation

The pilot is the team leader and is in overall charge of the aircraft and its occupants. The primary responsibility of the pilot and crew is to ensure the safety of the aircraft and its occupants. Their instructions must be obeyed. It is their decision whether to undertake the transfer or even to abort a mission and land at an unplanned destination. In an air ambulance undertaking an interfacility transport, there may be room for only one medical attendant. If present, an air ambulance paramedic will be available to assist, but he or she also has a role in assisting the pilot with communications and navigation.

C – communication

Lines of communication should be established for those retrieving or dispatching the patient, the aircrew and medical staff at the destination. The systematic approach to communication set out earlier in this book lends itself to the field of aviation transfer medicine because messages, often transmitted by radio, and through third parties, need to be succinct.

Named individuals and telephone numbers should be identified for liaison purposes. A central person or point of communication should be agreed where possible. Communication from aircraft is carried out by radio. Aircraft operational frequencies allow communication between the aircraft and civil or military airfields. In most cases it will not be possible to communicate directly with a land-based ambulance control centre, hospital switchboard or an emergency department.

> Communications are usually relayed, and must therefore be clear and concise and where possible should be through a single individual or point of contact.

Noise levels inside helicopters necessitate the use of headsets and microphones to communicate. Once on board, familiarisation with the headsets is a priority because this will be the primary method of communication during the transfer. At critical phases of flight (for example, takeoff and landing) the medical passengers and pilots will often all be 'connected'. At these times medical communication must be limited to the essentials. During the flight the medical passengers are often 'switched' on to a private channel where they can communicate without distracting the crew flying the aircraft. Some aircraft have satellite telephones or information can be relayed to the ground via the crew. Mobile phones should not be used on board aircraft.

Monitor alarms are difficult/impossible to hear, as is escaping gas from a cylinder that has been inadvertently switched on. It is advisable to divide up visual monitoring responsibilities where possible.

E – evaluation

The potential benefits of air transfer must be weighed against the risks:
- A hostile environment
- Very limited scope for medical intervention during flight
- Transfer by air may not shorten the duration of the journey if land-based vehicles must be used at each end
- It may be appropriate that competent patients/parents/guardians should be involved in the risk–benefit analysis so that their views can be taken into account.

> The decision to transfer by air rather than road should be given careful consideration and the views of the patient/parent/guardians taken into account.

P – preparation
Patient

The patient's physiological condition should be optimised as far as possible for the transfer. Access to the patient will be difficult in the confined aircraft environment where assessment and intervention are more challenging. Most helicopter air ambulances do not fly at heights greater than 1500 feet (500 m). At this height there is little reduction in barometric pressure, although trapped air will expand and there will be a small reduction in the partial pressure of oxygen.

Use the 'A, B, C, D, E' approach.

Airway

Security of the airway is particularly important given the multiple patient loading/unloading episodes. Endotracheal cuffs should be inflated with water rather than air to prevent cuff distension resulting in tracheal damage.

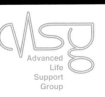

Breathing
Pneumothoraces require chest drains fitted with Heimlich valves. The reduction in partial pressure of oxygen (PO_2) at altitude may require an increase in fractional inspired oxygen concentration (FiO_2).

Circulation
A minimum of two points of intravenous access should be secured. Consider preparing boluses of fluid and inotrope infusions in advance (these may be difficult to prepare once under way). Fluid bags that contain any air may pressurise at altitude, resulting in a more rapid flow rate.

Disability
Intracranial air that may be present after a traumatic head injury will expand at altitude. It is recommended that these patients travel by air only in an aircraft pressurised to sea level.

Exposure
Ensure that patient temperature is maintained. Helicopters (especially military ones) can be quite cold.

Expansion
Remember that any trapped gas will expand at altitude, potentially causing pressure effects. Therefore nasogastric tubes should be kept on free drainage to deflate the stomach, and plaster casts should be 'bi-valved' if present.

Staff

Staff selected to undertake medical care in the air must be medically fit. An individual's propensity for motion, or air sickness, may influence the choice of personnel. Non-sedating prophylaxis in the form of medications such as cinnarizine can be instituted at a suitable interval before departure. Seabands, which are elasticated wristbands, acting on acupressure points could be considered as an alternative

Although little medical intervention can be achieved in flight, constant vigilance and care are required during the transportation to and from the aircraft. This requires competent and experienced medical staff. In addition, the Joint Aviation Authority requires that any staff assigned to travel in any aircraft must receive a briefing from the crew, including the location and operation of emergency exits, the use of communication equipment and specialist medical equipment, and the location and use of fire extinguishers (Appendix 1 to Joint Aviation Requirements of the UK Civil Aviation Authority – JAR OPS 3.005(d)).

Many UK air ambulances are able to carry only a maximum of two seated individuals, in addition to the pilot, although this figure may rise to three in some larger aircraft (Figure 14.1).

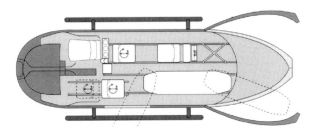

Fig. 14.1 EC 135 Helicopter configured for three 'passengers' and a stretcher. (Reproduced with permission from Bond Air Services UK.)

By contrast the military helicopters are not limited for space but may be cold and lighting tends to be poor.

P – packaging patient

Packaging the patient for an air transfer requires meticulous planning. As well as adopting the ABCDE approach as described in Chapter 6, additional thought must be given to the problems of air transport and, in particular, helicopter transfer.

Electrical equipment may emit electromagnetic radiation that could interfere with navigational or other onboard electrical systems. Any electronic medical equipment such as ventilators, monitors and syringe drivers that will be required for use in the aircraft must be approved by the Civil Aviation Authority (CAA). The approval has to specify the type and model of equipment, and the type and model of helicopter.

Most air ambulance services have some form of pre-hospital care ventilator and simple monitoring. Inevitably there will be several stages to the journey; equipment may have to be changed at each stage. Oxygen supplies on a helicopter are limited and you cannot easily stop to pick up more.

Part of the transfer process will inevitably mean that the patient is exposed to the elements and heat loss can be a problem.

In an air ambulance, there are often a limited number of headphones that allow communication. All passengers will require ear defenders of some sort. Conscious patients may find the sudden changes in noises and vibration, as when an air ambulance helicopter is about to land, frightening and this should be considered when headphones are in short supply.

Therapeutic equipment and supplies should be small and compact, easily securable and visible. All necessary drugs and equipment should be carried in an appropriately designed pack for ease of identification, preparation and use. A small case, or other stowage bag, should be taken in which to pack equipment for the return journey.

For helicopters, head, ear and eye protection will be required for both the patient and the team.

Staff

Accompanying personnel should carry the minimum personal equipment: a mobile telephone with useful telephone numbers, identification, some cash and a snack. Helicopter teams should wear protective goggles, a helmet, a flame-retardant flight suit and appropriate footwear. Ad hoc transport teams may have to improvise.

Transport back to base for personnel and equipment should be organised before the transfer is undertaken, because air ambulances and the RAF will return directly to their base airport, without giving medical staff a lift home.

> Close liaison with the air ambulance provider and the aircrew at all stages is vital in helping to understand the specific preparation and packaging requirements for air transfer.

T – transportation

The environment inside an aircraft has some unusual features. Most air ambulance designs have overcome some of the problems, but they are still cramped. Figure 14.1 shows an EC 135 helicopter configured for three 'passengers' and a stretcher.

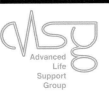

The main problems can be summarised as:
- Lack of manoeuvring space
- Lack of space for supplies
- Relatively noisy – staff may need to wear headphones to communicate
- Limited number of seats.

Military aircraft such as Sea King, Merlin and Chinooks are not limited for space. However, seating may be at more than an arm's length from the patient, making access difficult. Furthermore, because the aircraft has many functions and has not been specifically designed for the transfer of patients, there may be no purpose-built anchorage points for a stretcher. The ambient light is low, the noise level is high and the aircraft is cold; both staff and patients can suffer. Vibration can be disconcerting and makes visualisation of monitor screens difficult. A few moments spent arranging equipment, patient and personnel with the assistance and advice of the military crew is invaluable.

On helicopters, staff accompanying patients may be required to wear a safety helmet with built-in headphones or simply headphones. A heavy helmet makes head movement feel awkward, and the intercom sounds quiet and distant. When 'switched in' to the communications system, it is often difficult for the novice to ascertain who is talking to whom, and using the voice-operated microphone system is a skill in itself. The use of headphones and the noisy environment may render alarms on medical equipment inaudible. Equipment with visible alarm systems should be used if possible. End-tidal carbon dioxide monitoring is a valuable visual confirmation of ventilation in these circumstances.

Few hospitals are equipped with a helicopter landing area immediately outside their doors. It is therefore common for patients requiring transfer by air to be taken to the aircraft by a road vehicle, and delivered to hospital at their destination in the same way. Thus during transfer the patient will be moved to a new location several times. Each vehicle transfer represents a time of increased risk for the patient. Intravenous lines can be pulled out, ventilators can become disconnected and the medical team may be distracted. Care and good communication within the team are essential.

RETRIEVAL OF PATIENTS FROM HELICOPTERS

Most NHS staff will never actually transfer a patient in a helicopter; they are more likely to have to assist in the retrieval of a patient from a helicopter that has landed at their hospital. General guidelines for NHS trusts on their responsibilities for providing safety arrangements for landing helicopters are long overdue. Such guidelines should cover:
- Landing site preparation
- Retrieval team staff safety:
  - personal protective equipment
  - procedures.

Landing site preparation

Helicopters can land only at hospitals that have a purpose-built landing site, which must have been surveyed to the satisfaction of the air ambulance service operator. The hospital, or site operator, then has the responsibility to ensure that it keeps the site airworthy:
- Site operators should ensure vigilance in respect of building work, which may cause unidentified obstructions and hazards to landing aircraft.

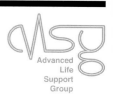

- Where possible the site should be inspected before every landing to ensure that the area is clear of debris. Items such as tin cans, paper and plastic sheeting can be sucked into the aircraft engine air intake, causing catastrophic engine failure; such debris can cause personal injury to ground retrieval team members.

- Site operators should ensure that a designated assembly point is identified, and positioned at a safe distance from the actual landing point. The assembly area should be positioned such that the team can clearly see the pilot and his or her hand signals.

- The road ambulance should be parked in a designated safe area; the vehicle should be positioned facing the aircraft in order to reduce the possibility that downdraft slams any open doors shut, trapping staff.

- All non-essential personnel and spectators must be kept away from the landing area and assembly point at all times during the operation. Particular care should be taken if children or animals are in the area. Hospital security and/or police officers should be available at the site. Security vigilance must be maintained until the helicopter has left the site and is well on its way.

- Fire and accidents are very rare; however, there is an increased risk of fire if the aircraft is being re-fuelled. Helicopter landing sites without immediate provision for fire fighting (equipment and trained personnel at the landing pad) will need to develop contingency plans with the local fire service.

Retrieval team staff safety

Personal protective equipment should be provided for, and used by, any staff who will be part of a retrieval team:

- High visibility (sunrise yellow or sunset red) jacket compliant with EN 471 – class 3
- Eye protection – preferably anti-misting goggles to be compliant with BS 166-345
- Ear defenders appropriate for the noise levels and anticipated frequencies and compliant with BS351-1
- Headgear may be considered as an optional extra, but should not interfere with the efficient fitting of ear protectors and eye protection.

In addition, footwear must be robust outdoor shoes; operating theatre clogs or high heels are not appropriate. Warm trousers should be worn; female staff must not wear dresses or skirts.

Approaching a helicopter

Only members of a ground retrieval team who have the specified personal protective equipment should be allowed to approach the helicopter. The team should position themselves in an assembly area from where they can see the helicopter and vice versa. No one on the ground should approach the aircraft until the pilot (or co-pilot) makes a clear hand signal to do so. If in doubt, wait. (In general, the crew of most air ambulances will send one of its crew members away from the aircraft to meet and escort the retrieval team towards the aircraft.)

The approach should be made from the front of the aircraft, keeping in full view of the pilot, initially, and later the crew member at the door to the aircraft. Never approach the helicopter from the rear. Tail rotor blades are lethal and may not be visible. If on a hill or sloping ground, approach and leave on the downhill side, in order to avoid the main rotor. Remember that, when stopped, the main rotor blades dip down towards the tip. If it becomes necessary to move from one

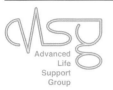

side of the aircraft to the other, having previously reached the fuselage, go around the nose and within arm's length of the aircraft.

Approach a helicopter
- Only when clearly instructed to do so
- In clear view of pilot

FIXED-WING AIR TRANSFERS

Most fixed-wing medical transfers are undertaken as a retrieval service by specialists; the international repatriation of sick or injured patients is a booming business. These repatriations require a great deal of forward planning, because flight slots have to be booked some time in advance. The repatriation teams often have to deal with different styles of health care in other countries as well as the problems of differing languages, which may lead to confusion.

When hospital staff are involved in the negotiations around the international repatriation of patients, it is important to record the following minimum contact details:
- The name of the repatriation company
- The contact person's name
- Telephone number (and fax number)
- The repatriation company's patient reference number
- The patient's name
- The patient's current location.

Some long distance air transfers involve the use of commercial airlines and the need to remove up to eight seats in an already overbooked flight. Aviation authorities, including the UK's CAA, usually strictly limit the carriage of any additional oxygen supplies on an aircraft.

SUMMARY

The information in this chapter is presented as an introduction only. Specialist air transfer training is not covered in detail either in this manual or on the PaNSTaR course. Further developments in conjunction with the STaR course are planned.

The safe transfer of patients by air requires an understanding of the benefits and limitations of this mode of transfer. Helicopter landings need to be undertaken under controlled conditions and safety is a paramount consideration. Understanding some of the problems of the international repatriation of patients may help receiving hospitals.

CHAPTER 15

Transfers and management of the child for scans in the radiology department

---

LEARNING OBJECTIVES

In this chapter you will learn about:
- Problems that are encountered during CT or MR scanning
- Solutions available to counteract these problems

INTRODUCTION

Sick infants and children commonly require complex radiological investigations. The transfer to and management of these children in the radiology department requires additional knowledge and skills above those needed for standard intra-hospital transfers. This chapter highlights the extra knowledge required.

THE RADIOLOGY DEPARTMENT

The department of radiology is historically an unsafe environment for ill children. In general the clinicians transferring the child will be unfamiliar with the layout and where anything is stored. Out of hours there will often be no clinical staff around from whom to seek help or advice. Each radiology department will differ from the others in which you have worked, so becoming familiar with these environments at an early stage is advised. The importance of familiarity with the environment is clearly recognised in the document *Provision of Anaesthetic Services in Magnetic Resonance Units* where it states:

> Only authorised personnel, who have received specific training and are fully conversant with the local safety rules, are allowed to enter the controlled area unsupervised.

In practice this means that you should not consider a transfer of any sort to such areas until you have been trained in the process and the environment.

In addition, scan rooms in radiology are a high workload area. The recurrent problem with such environments is that any problem leads to a rapidly escalating workload crisis. In such circumstances errors are common. Even those with a lot of experience in dealing with critically ill children may find themselves rapidly approaching overload in difficult circumstances. If a child deteriorates

---

Paediatric and Neonatal Safe Transfer and Retrieval: The Practical Approach, Edited by Steve Byrne, Steve Fisher, Peter-Marc Fortune, Cassie Lawn and Sue Wieteska. © 2008 Blackwell Publishing, ISBN: 978-1-4051-6919-6.

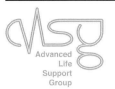

significantly it is often better to abandon the investigation and return at a later time rather than struggle with ongoing resuscitation in a hostile environment.

DIFFERENCES BETWEEN CT AND MR SCANS

The two scan modalities differ in their clinical indications, the information that they can provide and the hazards that they present. In general, CT (computed tomography) scans are useful for diagnosis of changes in bones, and for spotting large lumps or collections, and will give you this information rapidly. MR (magnetic resonance) scans are much slower, and have a range of different scan modes, which means that even a simple scan may take over half an hour (plus your organising time). It is not useful for looking at bony structures, but can differentiate within soft tissue structures, and can visualise the spinal cord and brain stem in detail despite the surrounding bone.

CT scanners work by means of scanning narrow beams of X-rays through the child, and measuring transmission. The X-ray source is rotated round the child, and the resulting data are summated into a two-dimensional section through the child. The scanning gantry may be angled in one plane only, and it is necessary to ensure that none of the transport equipment is damaged or disconnected by being caught by the gantry as it moves (Figure 15.1).

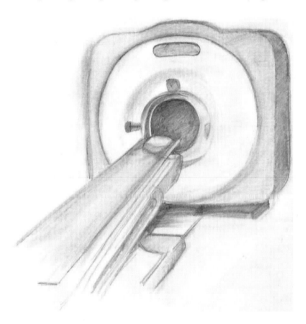

Fig. 15.1 CT scanner: vertical.

There is a potential radiation hazard to the transport staff resulting from these scanners. Any non-essential staff should be removed from the scan room during the scan. The number of essential staff in the scan room should be minimised and all those staying should be shielded. The indications for staff staying in the room are few and may include the need to hand ventilate a child, inability to read the data from the child's monitors from the control room or the need to restrain a moving child on a narrow plinth. Pregnant staff should not be present when radiation is used.

MR scanners work in a totally different way. At the core of the scanner is a large doughnut-shaped superconducting electromagnet, usually of 1–3 tesla (30 000–100 000 times the background magnetic field of the earth). Rotating protons (in body water) have a slight magnetic character, and line up with this field when the child is inserted into the centre of the scanner. Moving magnetic

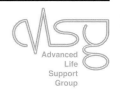

fields and radiofrequency energy that move protons out of alignment are applied to the child. When the applied energy is removed, the protons return to their ground state, giving up that energy, which can be measured by the sensing coils.

The child will be placed in the centre of the scanner, which will completely envelop most children, making them inaccessible and largely lost from view.

At present there are no data to show that there is a health risk to staff from these levels of exposure to either static or moving magnetic fields, or from the radiofrequency energy. However, a European guideline has been proposed for exposure limits that would prevent staff staying in the scan room during the scan should it be introduced unmodified at the proposed date of 2008. In general pregnant staff should avoid the scan room where possible, particularly in the first trimester.

TRANSFER TO AND FROM THE RADIOLOGY DEPARTMENT

For transport to the scan area, the child should be on an appropriate transfer trolley or bed with the transport equipment attached. An appropriate level of monitoring must be established, and oxygen and battery supplies must be sufficient for the transfer to the scanner and back with a reasonable reserve. If there is not a wall oxygen supply it is essential that you have an MRI-compatible oxygen cylinder sufficient for the scan time. The child must be accompanied by staff who are trained appropriately, and capable of managing circulatory and airway problems en route. Drugs and equipment to permit this should be carried. Sedation or anaesthesia, if appropriate, should be continued to maintain child comfort.

SPECIFIC PROBLEMS PRESENTED BY CROSS-SECTIONAL SCANNERS

CT scanner

Key problems presented by the CT scanner are listed in Box 15.1. In essence, CT scans require a still child, are often very quick (a matter of a few minutes), and do not usually pose major problems of access to or monitoring of the child.

> **Box 15.1 Problems and requirements of a CT scan**
>
> - Unfamiliar environment
> - Isolated site
> - Time-limited slots
> - Relatively short time required
> - Immobile child

With a stable, breathing infant, you need to make a decision before going to scan whether they are likely to remain still for the period of the scan. A feed just before a scan in well infants may encourage sleep and thus a still child, but precludes anaesthesia.

In sick or unstable younger children or where more complex CT scans are required, sedation or anaesthesia may be required. Where control of the airway is needed, it should be undertaken only by those familiar with these procedures and the radiology environment.

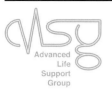

In those children requiring ventilatory support, gas tubing and all monitoring leads to be used must be long enough for movement of the child in the scanner. There is no reason why the gas supplies, ventilator and monitors from the transport module cannot be used throughout the scan. However, it is recommended that, as most CT scan rooms have piped oxygen and many have piped air, the transport unit should be transferred onto the gas and power supplies present in the scan room to conserve the capacity of the cylinders.

MR scanner

The MR scanner is probably the most difficult environment inside or outside a hospital to care for a sick child safely. The key problems posed are listed in Box 15.2.

Box 15.2 Additional problems associated with an MRI environment

- Very poor access to child
- Very hostile to staff (health, implants, noise level)
- Very hostile to child (minimal access, claustrophobia, noise)
- Incompatible with standard monitoring equipment
- Incompatible with continuous infusion devices
- Incompatible with routine ventilators and gas bottles
- Immobile child
- Relatively long duration of scans necessitates airway control ± ventilation

---

The scans take much longer to do than CT scans – each component of the scan takes 3–7 min to acquire all the necessary information. In total, scan times in excess of 40 min are common. The child must therefore be immobile during this period, and appropriate sedation or general anaesthesia may be necessary to ensure a satisfactory scan. Although the scan is not painful, the effect of the gradient magnetic field is such that there is significant pulsatile background noise (up to 95 dB(A) for 1.5 tesla magnet). This can be quite frightening, so ear protection is necessary.

The MRI environment

The key problem is safety. The presence of a very, very powerful magnet means that no ferromagnetic objects are permitted in the MR scan room, which includes most of what you brought down with you – conventional gas cylinders, ventilators, normal trolleys, laryngoscopes, many syringe drivers and most monitoring equipment. Gas cylinders introduced into the scan room have been pulled out of hands into the scanner, and have resulted in the death of a child being scanned. A brief search of the internet will produce lots of images of large, solid objects being pulled into the magnet.

The radiographer in charge of the scanner has absolute authority with regard to management of this problem for very sound reasons. If there is a problem, assume that you are wrong, because you almost certainly will be! No one will be allowed into the scan room until it has been established that it is safe for them to enter. Some people with implants (including pacemakers) or foreign bodies in soft tissues may never be permitted into the scan room. All pockets should be emptied, and keys, coins, badges, wallets, watches, stethoscopes, etc. removed and left outside the scan room. Credit cards are wiped by the magnets! Hair grips and clips are a lesser problem, but are best removed where reasonable. Glasses, belt buckles and metal components of clothes and underwear are not a problem for staff, although a tug may be felt if that person moves close to the magnet. The static magnetic field is always present, although it may be switched off (or quenched) in an emergency. As quenching the magnet this way requires weeks to restore it to normal function again, at very considerable cost, this is acceptable only for immediate threat to life or limb.

The child will be subjected to the same scrutiny as the staff, but it will be applied more rigidly. Any metal will distort the magnetic field to some degree and impair the scan of the region around that metal. This will include all one-way valves sometimes found in airway or vascular access devices. All attached medical aids must be considered. Shiley tracheostomy tubes are safe; Bivona tracheostomy tubes contain a metal coil and are not. Where possible all non-compatible equipment should be removed, or secured as far away from the region to be scanned as possible. ECG leads and electrodes, and pulse oximeter probes, should be removed. Start at the head end and visualise every inch of your child to ensure that all such devices have been removed. Moving magnetic fields and radiofrequency energy induce electrical currents in anything metallic or conductive. If a metallic object is missed, this may result in localised heating, and possible skin burns.

The MR scanner is a long narrow tunnel. Once inside the scanner it is almost impossible to get near the child. The combination of very poor access to the child, the claustrophobia and sheer noisiness of the environment, and the need for absolutely still children for a prolonged period means that most children will require general anaesthesia and airway and ventilatory control.

Airway and breathing

If your child is not already intubated or the airway controlled, this will need to be undertaken before entering the MR scanner. If your child is already ventilated, it is still not safe to enter the scan room. An appropriate, MRI-compatible ventilator is necessary, which may be part of the equipment in the scan room or may be taken there with you. The ventilator must be capable of operating on the gas supplies available in the scan room. Oxygen is universally available, but piped air is not always present. Although some MRI-compatible, non-ferrous cylinders are available for use as a reserve, they are small and very expensive, and many units have chosen to eliminate all cylinders from the scan room to eliminate the possibility of a non-compatible cylinder being introduced in error. If your transport ventilator is MRI compatible, it must be capable of being removed from the transport trolley and taken into the scan room. In this case a second child ventilation circuit is essential to support the child during the period without the mechanical ventilator. In some hospitals the only ventilation equipment is based around an MRI-compatible anaesthetic machine. Use of such equipment without appropriate experience is extremely hazardous. In these circumstances all ventilated children should be managed by an experienced anaesthetist familiar with the local set-up.

Monitoring in the MRI environment

MRI-compatible monitoring is available in some units but is very expensive, and what is available in your hospital may not conform to normal recommended monitoring standards. ECG may be recorded using MRI-compatible electrodes and either appropriately shielded or carbon fibre cables, with fibreoptic connections to the base monitor. Normal ECG electrodes and cables are highly dangerous

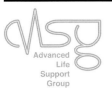

and should never be used because of the large amounts of energy generated in the ECG leads, resulting in skin burns, and the distortion of the magnetic field from metal components in the ECG electrodes. Pulse oximetry uses fibreoptic cables to direct light to the child and back to the photodetectors. Non-invasive blood pressure uses familiar technology, but needs to avoid metal connectors. Invasive arterial blood pressure monitoring is available in some units.

The electronics of the base unit need careful screening from the effects of the scanner environment, and there may be specific limits as to where the monitors can be placed. Often the power supplies have greater restrictions than the monitor itself. If anaesthetics are given in the MR scanner, oxygen and carbon dioxide monitoring must be available. Current recommendations are that there should be monitor screens both in the scan room itself and in the adjacent control room, so that the child can be monitored without the immediate presence of the staff.

Medications by infusion in the scan room

If children are on infusions, these should be discontinued where possible. At this point there are no MRI-compatible syringe drivers widely available, because of the metal components in the motor and the magnetic principle by which the motor works. Attempts to use these in MR scanners have resulted in the syringe driver becoming a missile, or the motor reversing under the influence of the scanner. If it is necessary to continue an infusion, consideration should be given to postponing the scan, or seeking alternative diagnostic tests. It is possible to set up a second syringe driver in the control room (outside the scan room itself). The line is then run with three or four extension lines through a waveguide (a narrow tube that passes through the protective wall surrounding the scanner) to the child. The infusion can be swapped over to this new one and the child stabilised before being taken into the scan room. This does add substantially to the complexity of what is already a highly complex operation and is inadvisable where infusions, such as inotropes, are critical to child stability.

Temperature control

It is difficult to be specific about temperature changes in children undergoing an MR scan. Although the magnet is cooled by liquid helium, and the scan room is very well ventilated, the scan also puts a lot of energy into the tissues being scanned. A safety limit is based on the child's weight to avoid excessive heating. This can result either in a degree of cooling or warming depending on the precise scan, with a degree of warming (up to 0.5°C in small babies) being more common. It is probably simpler to avoid extremes and cover the child with a moderately warm cover.

Emergencies

In the event of a major problem in the MR scanner the priority should normally be to move the child out of the scan room before attempting to manage the specifics of the problem. Although simple airway problems may respond to adjustments without needing to remove the child, none of the equipment that you will need to diagnose or treat the problem is likely to be safe to bring into the scan room. In the event of a cardiac arrest, the arrival of the cardiac arrest team with arrest trolley is likely to pose more of a hazard to the child and transport staff than provide any useful help.

SUMMARY

The provision of safe and effective transport and care to, from and in the radiology department in general (and the MR scan room in particular) poses major problems to both the child and the attending medical carers. It should be undertaken only by those with specific training in the major hazards that it poses.

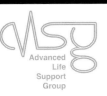

CHAPTER 16

Transporting the child with a difficult airway

LEARNING OBJECTIVES

In this chapter you will learn about:
- How and when to transport unintubated children
- How to assess and approach children with potentially difficult airways

---

INTRODUCTION

When there is any doubt about the security of a child's airway the safest option will usually be to intubate before transfer. However, there are a number of exceptions to this rule and there are also times where it may be foreseen that intubation will be extremely challenging. These scenarios are discussed below.

During the initial assessment phase of a transfer it is vital that clinicians consider the status of the child's airway. The transport consultant should be immediately alerted if there is any airway compromise, especially if there are reasons to suspect that intubation may be difficult or that it would be better to transport the child unintubated. Very careful consideration should be given to selecting the team who undertake such transfers; they must have sufficient skills to package and transfer the child with the minimum of risk and be capable of intervening en route if it becomes necessary. It is unlikely that it is ever appropriate to mobilise junior members of the transport team on these occasions.

Many of the children described above might be classified as HDU (high dependency unit) children. These children are frequently transferred in the UK by clinicians who have not received extensive ICU (intensive care unit) or transport training. In other countries such as Australia most of them will be transported by an ICU transport team. In either case the key to safe management is careful consideration of the factors at play in each case, deployment of the best available team and an avoidance of underestimating the problems that may be encountered.

Where the issue is primarily of difficult intubation, there may be expertise in the referring centre's anaesthetic department to assist either the referring or the transferring team. This may enable resolution of the acute situation. If that expert is not going to travel with the child the consultant in charge of the transfer is responsible for deciding that it is safe to continue with the transfer.

Paediatric and Neonatal Safe Transfer and Retrieval: The Practical Approach, Edited by Steve Byrne, Steve Fisher, Peter-Marc Fortune, Cassie Lawn and Sue Wieteska. © 2008 Blackwell Publishing, ISBN: 978-1-4051-6919-6.

THE UNINTUBATED CHILD

Unintubated children will usually be fully conscious and may be fairly mobile. Any compromise that they have to their upper airway is likely to worsen if they become upset or agitated. It is usually preferable that a parent travel with the child in such situations because they are likely to be the best person to keep the child calm. In these circumstances the accompanying parent effectively becomes a part of the transfer team. They should be briefed both on what to expect and on what is expected of them. An advance agreement should be established with the parent that they shall vacate the immediate clinical area should a crisis occur. In an ambulance this might be achieved by them sitting in the cab with the driver/paramedic while the vehicle is parked up and the situation resolved.

DIFFICULT INTUBATION

Difficult intubation may arise as an expected or unexpected event. True unexpected difficult intubation occurs in 3% of adult elective anaesthetic practice and is thought to be less common in paediatric practice.

PREDICTION OF DIFFICULT VENTILATION

There are a number of factors that should alert clinicians to the possibility of a difficult airway. An inability to place the child's head in the ideal intubation position (neutral for a baby or sniffing the morning air for an older child) can result in a suboptimal view at laryngoscopy. In some conditions the child's neck may be fixed in a suboptimal position as the result of disease. Also some children may have potentially unstable necks that preclude excessive (or any) manipulation of their head position (trauma, achondroplasia). In these situations, the limited anatomical extension of the head on the neck means that the child's head cannot be put into the ideal intubation position. Lack of mouth opening and reduced mobility of the mandible may also predict difficult intubation.

Mallampati's scores can be useful in the adult population during preoperative anaesthetic assessment. This test may be difficult in children because it requires them to cooperate but it can be very useful. The Mallampati score is assessed by viewing the posterior part of the pharynx, with the child in the sitting position and looking straight ahead with the mouth wide open. The child should not say 'Aah' during the test because this elevates the soft palate and gives a false impression of the score (Figure 16.1).

Children who have been previously intubated should have a record of that procedure including a grading of the ease of intubation based on a system by Lehane and McCormick (Figure 16.2). Although this may not be recorded in all cases, it will usually be found where signs that might predict difficulty at intubation are present. It is important to note that an inexperienced clinician may not be able to obtain the same views as an experienced anaesthetist or intensivist.

CLASSIFICATION OF DIFFICULT AIRWAY SCENARIOS

1 Predicted difficult intubation with known easy mask ventilation
2 Predicted difficult intubation with mask ventilation of unknown efficacy
3 Unpredicted difficult intubation with easy mask ventilation

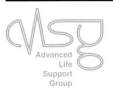

4 Unpredicted difficult intubation with where the child is difficult or impossible to ventilate
5 Upper airway obstruction.

Each of these situations may occur in a child with a full stomach, which needs to be considered in the approach to the airway.

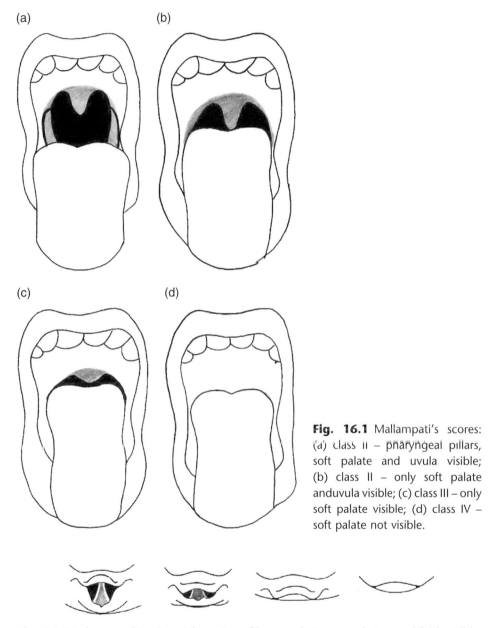

Fig. 16.1 Mallampati's scores: (a) class II – pharyngeal pillars, soft palate and uvula visible; (b) class II – only soft palate anduvula visible; (c) class III – only soft palate visible; (d) class IV – soft palate not visible.

Fig. 16.2 Lehane and McCormick scoring of laryngeal views: grade I – vocal folds visible; grade II – arytenoids cartilages and posterior part of vocal folds visible; grade III – epiglottis visible; grade IV – epiglottis not visible.

GENERAL PREPARATION FOR DIFFICULT INTUBATION

The transport team should always carry extra equipment appropriate to their child group to deal with an unexpected difficult intubation:

• Bougie
• Stylet

• Smaller tubes
• Different laryngoscopes, for example, McCoy, straight blade, polio blade.
Difficulty in intubation may result from an inability to visualise the larynx, an inability to pass the tube through the larynx or a combination of both. Failure to view the larynx may be resolved by repositioning the airway or manipulation of the larynx into view by the laryngoscopist or his or her assistant. The standard first manipulation may be remembered by the 'BURP' mnemonic: 'back, upwards, right and press'. This indicates the usual direction of force required to improve the view at laryngoscopy.

Stylets and gum elastic bougies are aids to intubation and no retrieval team should travel without an appropriate range of sizes.

Gum elastic bougies

These come in three sizes: 5 Ch, 10 Ch and 15 Ch. The smallest size (5 Ch) passes though a 2.5 mm endotracheal (ET) tube. The bougie may be placed through the vocal folds and the ET tube may then be railroaded over it. The bougie is particularly useful in the situation where the view of the larynx is less than ideal and the larynx is anterior or pushed to one side. The narrow bougie is much easier to place in the larynx than an ET tube. The smallest bougies have a rigid end and therefore may cause trauma to the airway; gentle use is essential.

Note that when the ET tube is railroaded it may become caught on the arytenoid cartilages posteriorly or the vocal folds laterally. A twisting motion as the tube passes into the larynx often allows such an obstacle to be overcome.

Stylets

These are available for all sizes of ET tubes. A stylet is used to stiffen the ET tube, which allows the tube to be directed towards the larynx more easily. The stylet should *never* be allowed to protrude from the distal end of the ET tube because it may traumatise or perforate the trachea.

PREDICTED DIFFICULT INTUBATION

If time allows a senior anaesthetist with advanced airway skills and an experienced assistant should be present. Preparation should be made with availability of a full range of equipment for difficult intubation. This would include light wands and fibreoptic intubating equipment.

Anaesthesia for the known difficult intubation should aim to maintain spontaneous respiration until the ET tube is placed securely in the larynx.

FAILED INTUBATION WHERE VENTILATION IS POSSIBLE

In anaesthetic practice the approach in the failed intubation, where ventilation is possible, is to wake the child. This is unlikely to be practical in the intensive care scenario but should be considered. If ventilation can be maintained, repeated attempts to intubate are unlikely to result in success and an alternative strategy should be used.

The assistance of an experienced anaesthetist and an ENT (ear, nose and throat) surgeon should be sought simultaneously. An experienced anaesthetist may be able to perform a successful intubation using direct laryngoscopy or may need to perform fibreoptic intubation. If intubation proves impossible emergency tracheostomy may be needed.

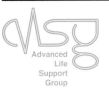

FAILED INTUBATION WHERE VENTILATION IS IMPOSSIBLE

Difficulty in intubation may be associated with serious complications. A failure to intubate may be managed provided that it is possible to ventilate the child's lungs. Failure to ventilate creates a life-threatening situation and requires timely and effective action to ensure ventilation by means other than bag – valve – mask. If this occurs the following strategies should be employed:

1 Don't panic! The first rule of the 'can't intubate, can't ventilate situation' is to get help and keep calm. In district general hospitals, there may be a senior anaesthetist who should be fast bleeped to attend and assist.

2 Bag – valve – mask ventilate: initial attempts to ventilate should include re-positioning the airway with maximum jaw thrust. Additional help should be sought to facilitate a good facemask seal and bag ventilation. An oropharyngeal airway and a nasopharyngeal airway should be tried.

3 Laryngeal mask airway: if there is failure to oxygenate using the bag–valve–mask, a laryngeal mask should be inserted. A maximum of two attempts should be made to site the laryngeal mask.

4 Cricothyroidotomy: if there is still failure to oxygenate at this point it is neces-sary to perform a needle cricothyroidotomy for children aged <8 years old and a surgical cricothyroidotomy for those >8 years (for further details see *Advanced Paediatric Life Support: The Practical Approach* – ALSG 2005).

UPPER AIRWAY OBSTRUCTION

Croup and subglottic stenosis are the most common reasons for upper airway obstruction in children. Epiglottitis has become less common since Hib immunisa-tion was introduced.

The recommended technique in upper airway obstruction is to maintain spon-taneous ventilation during induction of anaesthesia. Gaseous induction with halothane or sevoflurane in oxygen may be used. Spontaneous respiration does not always maintain oxygenation; continuous positive airway pressure (CPAP) may be required via the anaesthetic breathing circuit as anaesthesia deepens. On occasion apnoea may occur at deep levels of anaesthesia, especially in small babies.

In upper airway obstruction the view of the larynx may be difficult to obtain because of abnormal anatomy or swelling of normal structures. There may also be anatomical abnormalities below the level of the vocal folds that make passage of the ET tube difficult (even if the view is normal at laryngoscopy).

Croup and subglottic stenosis narrow the airway at the level of the cricoid ring below the vocal folds. The larynx itself may look completely normal. Difficulty is experienced in passing the ET tube beyond the level of the vocal folds into the upper trachea. When the tube is passed through the vocal folds the obstruction is felt and it is not possible to advance the tube further. A smaller tube should be chosen and a gentle rotating movement used to advance the tube. It may be necessary to use a tube several sizes smaller than originally planned. In larger children special 'croup tubes' will be required. These are longer than standard tubes, and are cut to a length suitable for the smaller children in whom they are usually used. Care should be taken not to cause trauma and make the narrowing worse. A rotational movement at the tip of the ET tube may facilitate a round tube moving through the funnel-shaped entrance formed by the vocal folds and the narrower cricoid ring below.

When the cricoid ring is narrowed it may be useful to use an ET tube that has been kept cold in the refrigerator. This prevents buckling of the soft tube when gentle forward pressure is applied to take the tube through the narrowing. Holding the tip of the tube with a pair of Magill's forceps, about 3 cm from the end, allow the tip to be guided more precisely. The aperture through the cricoid ring may not line up with the centre of the aperture of the larynx. This offset means that repeated attempts to place the tube through the centre of the vocal folds may not be successful. Gentle rotation towards the anterior and posterior of the larynx may find the aperture through the larynx.

SUMMARY

The child with a difficult airway presents some of the most challenging problems encountered in paediatric transport medicine. It is vital that at all times the consultant in charge be fully appraised of the situation so that he or she can ensure that appropriate support is provided to minimise the risks involved. For those delivering the transport care careful planning must cover both prevention of, and strategies to deal with, the potential complications that can be anticipated. Experience and an ability to remain calm in stressful situations are essential.

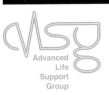

CHAPTER 17

Keeping safe in the transport environment

LEARNING OBJECTIVES

In this chapter you will learn about:
- The importance of keeping the medical team safe during transfer
- The importance of keeping the child safe during a transfer
- The importance of minimising the danger to the general public during a transfer

---

Safely transporting a critically ill child requires a coordinated approach. The transport environment is hazardous. Travelling in the rear compartment of a road ambulance is fraught with potential danger.

This chapter focuses on safety in the transport environment in terms of:
- transfer team members
- the child
- the parents
- equipment
- the ambulance
- speed.

TRANSFER TEAM MEMBERS

Clothing

All staff should prepare for the worst. It is never possible to predict whether an ambulance is likely to break down, so adequate clothing should always be carried to ensure sufficient protection against the weather. Proprietary reflective jackets or vests should be provided for all staff to ensure good visibility if they have to step outside the ambulance while parked at the roadside. Shoes should be appropriate for the roadside environment; theatre clogs are not suitable for undertaking external transfers.

Manual handling

All personnel undertaking transfers should have received training in manual handling. Transfers are often undertaken in cramped conditions and may involve movement of heavy children and equipment into and out of ambulances and other vehicles. These movements present a significant risk to the health of

---

Paediatric and Neonatal Safe Transfer and Retrieval: The Practical Approach, Edited by Steve Byrne, Steve Fisher, Peter-Marc Fortune, Cassie Lawn and Sue Wieteska. © 2008 Blackwell Publishing, ISBN: 978-1-4051-6919-6.

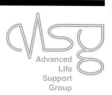

transfer personnel. A risk assessment by your trust manual handling services may identify some useful ways of reducing this risk. Whether or not this is undertaken, each team member is responsible for assessing the risks both to themselves and to others.

Where possible automated equipment should be used (for example, tail lifts) and loose equipment packed into specially designed trolleys. If these facilities are not available, use stretcher trolleys or wheelchairs to transport equipment. Do not hesitate to ask for help from local staff when required.

Established teams should examine their transport kit and pursue modifications that may improve manual handling characteristics. Always use a Patslide or other aid to move larger children between stretchers.

Be careful: the transport environment is not kind to backs!

Infection control

Medical staff should have received full immunisation against hepatitis B. Never compromise on the use of standard precautions. Hand hygiene should not be forgotten and gloves, plastic apron, mask/face shield/goggles should always be used as they would be on the ward.

It is best practice always to assume that the child is infectious and behave accordingly, because it is uncommon for microbiology results to be available before the departure of the transport team.

Be especially careful with bodily fluids, including respiratory secretions when suctioning. Always wear a surgical mask and eye protection, or use a closed system.

Where there is a suspicion of especially virulent and highly infectious aetiology special precautions must be taken. These include double gloving/gown/goggles/ N95 mask or filtering facepiece respirator, or powered air-purifying respirator (PAPR) as appropriate. Only those trained and regularly updated in their use should wear these types of personal protective equipment (PPE). For further information, consult the Health Protection Agency (www.hpa.org.uk) (see Chapter 18).

Sharps

The potential to sustain a sharps injury during the resuscitation and stabilisation of a critically ill child, in unfamiliar territory, such as another hospital or the back of an ambulance, is higher than in a practitioner's usual place of work. Be extra vigilant. Find out where the sharps bin is and ensure that your sharps are immediately disposed of. Be watchful of others and do not injure yourself on someone else's sharps.

Ensure that the transfer vehicle that you use has an easily accessible sharps bin. All syringes that are preloaded for the journey should be capped off with needleless caps, not sheathed syringe needles.

Restraint

All staff travelling in an ambulance or other vehicle must wear seatbelts while the vehicle is in motion. If interventions are required that cannot be performed by a team member when in the seated, belted position, the vehicle must be stopped.

Wherever possible team members should be seated such that they have access to the child and an adequate view of the monitors. Access to infusion pumps and infusion lines for bolus fluids should also be possible.

> An unrestrained team member becomes a missile in a collision.

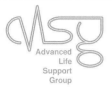

THE CHILD

Clothing

Heat loss through convection, conduction and radiation is all increased in the transfer environment. Careful wrapping of the child to minimise heat loss, without compromising access for clinical observations and interventions, can be very difficult. The use of foil thermal wraps, vacuum mattresses and the BabyPOD can all help in this regard. If using a vacuum mattress with a heating gel pack small children may become overheated. The child's temperature should be measured regularly.

Where a child is fully anaesthetised, exposure when moving between vehicles may be minimised by completely covering the child for a brief time. If you do use this method, it is important to be explicit about your intentions to ensure that no one interprets the covering as a signal of death!

Infection control

Critically ill children may have impaired immunity. It is important not to compromise on sterile technique when inserting or accessing lines, drains or catheters during a transfer.

Restraint

Over the body 'cross-straps', provided as standard on most ambulance stretchers, provide very little restraint in the horizontal plane. Currently commercially available 'over-the-shoulder' adjustable five-point harnesses are not available for all sizes of baby or child. The new infant neorestraint can be used for all sizes of infant, although it requires an adjustment of existing transport incubators to allow its use. There is therefore no definitive solution at the current time. A number of companies are said to be working in this area and it is hoped that a wider range of solutions should be available in the near future. In the meantime, an awareness that child restraint needs to be as effective as possible is likely to ensure the best possible use of the available resource.

PARENTS

Clothing

If parents accompany the transport team it is important that they have appropriate clothing and footwear for all eventualities as described above for the staff.

Restraint

When travelling in the ambulance, parents must always wear the seatbelt provided. It must be made clear that they must not release it unless the ambulance has come to a halt and the transport team and/or driver has instructed the parent that it is safe to do so.

EQUIPMENT

Manual handling

General issues of manual handling are discussed above; equipment should be assembled into bags or boxes, which ideally wheel along but may be carried if that is not possible. Once again your trust manual handling department may be helpful with the design of kit that meets the needs of the team with minimisation of manual handling risk.

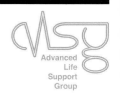

Infection control

All equipment should be clean and uncontaminated. Use breathing system filters to protect the child and the ventilator. An appropriate maintenance/cleaning schedule for all equipment should be adhered to.

Restraint

Unrestrained equipment becomes a missile when sudden deceleration occurs during a collision. All equipment, no matter how small and insignificant, must be restrained. Established retrieval teams should ensure that it is possible to secure all their equipment into the back of the ambulance, in compliance with CEN guidelines (see below).

For adhoc teams a compromise using over the top 'cross-straps' on the ambulance stretcher may be useful to restrain equipment. Most ambulances also have appropriate restraints for portable oxygen bottles, but, if not, make sure that they are put away in cupboards or strapped down firmly elsewhere.

AMBULANCE

The CEN (European Committee for Standardisation) standard for ambulances in the UK (BS EN 1789:2000 – Medical Vehicles and their Equipment – Road Ambulances) is voluntary. The Vehicle Certification Agency (www.vca.gov.uk) provides certificates of CEN compliance, and most ambulance providers are ensuring that newly purchased vehicles are CEN certified.

It is notable that equipment not normally carried in the ambulance is exempt from this regulation and also the restraint of children in the rear compartment of the ambulance is not regulated. Despite this, everyone involved in transfers should seek out the best possible solutions for both their own and the child's safety.

Manual handling

Ambulance crews are used to manual handling and are a useful resource. Hydraulic lifts should be used wherever provided to load and unload stretchers, incubators and equipment.

For stability most stretchers should be moved only when at their lowest position to prevent tipping – this means that extendable handles need to be used to manoeuvre the stretcher.

Infection control

Cleaning schedules for ambulance interiors should be adhered to and documented as per, for example, the Joint Royal Colleges Ambulance Liaison Committee (JRCALC guidelines).

A sharps bin should be available within the ambulance – make sure that it is within reach if it is required during the journey.

Restraint

As above, all passengers must use seatbelt restraints where fitted – preferably a full three-point harness. No one should stand up while the ambulance is moving: always ask the driver to stop first.

When you board the vehicle have a look at the interior and note the position of the fixtures and fittings. If anyone is unrestrained in the rear of the ambulance, he or she may become a missile, and the projecting fittings are areas with which they will collide. Other occupants will also be endangered by an unrestrained passenger. Think about where staff sit; if you are unable to restrain the child

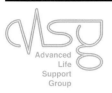

adequately, the rearward facing seat at the child's head should be used only if there is no alternative.

If you are fortunate enough to have a purpose-built vehicle for transfers, make sure that the cupboards can be used to store your equipment and that there are clamps for all equipment necessary for transfer (ventilator/pumps, etc.).

SPEED

There is often a sense of urgency about transport of the critically ill child to intensive care, which may lead to the use of lights and sirens and emergency driving techniques on both outbound and inbound journeys. There is evidence that the risks of collision are increased during journeys where lights and sirens and exemptions (such as speeding, passing through red lights) are used.

The acceleration and deceleration forces associated with this sort of driving technique are increased and may affect the team in terms of their comfort and ability to perform their duties. Furthermore the child may be compromised by reduced physiological stability. This is especially true in the preterm infant.

Travelling using lights and sirens and exemptions over long distances is more stressful and tiring for the driver and may be harmful for the child. For all these reasons, emergency driving techniques are not normally necessary or desirable.

Strategies to reduce the need for emergency driving techniques:
• Promote a culture of safety over speed
• Use telephone advice to support local resources in the resuscitation and stabilisation of the child
• Reduce transport team mobilisation time
• Ensure destination and route are confirmed before departure
• Prepare the child for stable transfer
• Pursue a system of smooth progress with the traffic
• Use clinical triage to stratify urgency and inform driving techniques.

Convoys of blue light vehicles are more dangerous than a single vehicle; for this reason, in some parts of the country the police do not provide police escorts to ambulances.

Do not use excessive speed or cross red lights unless absolutely necessary.

SUMMARY

Transport of the critically ill child aims to provide safe transfer from the referring to the receiving centre. This requires a multidisciplinary approach with an emphasis on a culture of safety.

Special attention should be paid to the fixation of everything that goes in the back of the ambulance: staff, child and equipment.

Excessive road speed and use of exemptions should be considered only in exceptional circumstances.

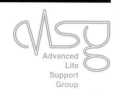

CHAPTER 18

The infectious or contaminated child

LEARNING OBJECTIVE

In this chapter you will learn about:

- The essential differences between infectious and chemically contaminated children
- A structured approach to the safe management of the infectious child
- How to assess the risk of a child being infectious
- How the principles of ACCEPT can assist safe transfers
- Some information about chemical contamination

INTRODUCTION

There is currently a heightened awareness of the risks of the transmission of infection both to staff and between children. Infectious children may pose a threat to others until the infection is eradicated. During a hospital admission, an infectious child may require transfer within the hospital or even to a specialist centre in another hospital. Such transfers expose healthcare workers to the ongoing risk of infection transmission.

Contaminated children are usually those who have been exposed to some form of chemical released as a result of an accidental spillage outside the hospital. Such children pose a threat only to those who come into close physical contact. Once properly decontaminated, the threat disappears and it becomes safe to transfer these children according to their medical needs.

In all situations involving children extra vigilance must be employed to ensure the safety of the immediate family. Where parents or relatives have not been exposed to the risk agent they must not be allowed to come into contact with the child without appropriate precautions. This exception to normal practice is likely to be difficult to enforce and may upset both the child and their relatives, but is essential to prevent the creation of further casualties.

THE POTENTIALLY INFECTIOUS CHILD

Standard Precautions, or what used to be called 'Universal Precautions', should remind healthcare staff that all children should be regarded as potential sources of infections, which may be transmitted to the staff or between children.

Paediatric and Neonatal Safe Transfer and Retrieval: The Practical Approach, Edited by Steve Byrne, Steve Fisher, Peter-Marc Fortune, Cassie Lawn and Sue Wieteska. © 2008 Blackwell Publishing, ISBN: 978-1-4051-6919-6.

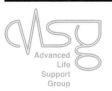

The transfer of the infectious or contaminated child is usually a primary transfer, performed by the ambulance service, from a residence, or the scene of an incident, to the hospital's Emergency Department. However, once admitted, such children may need to undergo a secondary transfer to another hospital, where tertiary specialist care is available. If not transferred out, infectious children will still have to be transferred safely within the hospital from the Emergency Department to an appropriate location within the hospital.

> When dealing with cases of unusual illness, which may be infectious or as a result of contamination, the welfare of staff and other children is paramount; the emphasis is on prevention of transmission.

An ABCD approach to the safety aspects of infection control may be used. To avoid confusion and for the purposes of this book, these will be referred to in lower case (a, b, c, d) as in Table 18.1, linking this in with the ACCEPT structure.

Table 18.1 The a, b, c, d approach to the safety aspects of infection control

	Title	Description
a	alert	Be alert to the possibility of transmissible disease
b	barrier	Use barrier precautions (physical separation and personal protective equipment or PPE)
c	clean and disinfect	Ensure that all potentially contaminated equipment and surfaces are cleaned and disinfected
d	dispose	Ensure safe handling and disposal of all waste

A – ASSESSMENT

- What is the problem?
- What is being/should be done?
- What is the effect of these actions?
- What is needed next?

The problem is that any child may pose an infection risk. Following the outbreak of severe acute respiratory syndrome (SARS) and concerns about the possibility of the epidemic spread of severe flu-like viral infections, there is a general state of heightened awareness of the possibility of an epidemic of life-threatening viral respiratory illnesses. Staff in Emergency Departments are advised to be 'a' (alert) to the possibility that a child presenting with unusual illness may be the index case for an outbreak.

The following enquiries should be made:
- Where has the child been recently?
- Where does the child live?
- Where does the child go to school/playgroup?
- Has the child travelled abroad?
- How did the child travel?

Mechanisms are in place to alert those in the front line to any emerging pattern of increases in reported infections. The Health Protection Agency (HPA) is charged with coordinating health protection across the UK. The Communicable Disease Surveillance Centre (CDSC), which is part of the HPA, receives information and coordinates the dissemination of surveillance intelligence. Other sources of information include Euro surveillance; weekly updates are distributed as *Communicable Disease Report Weekly* (CDR Weekly). If necessary alerts are emailed to key personnel in hospital and primary care trusts. In effect the HPA acts as a barometer of the spread of infectious diseases, not only in the UK but also anywhere in the world (Figure 18.1).

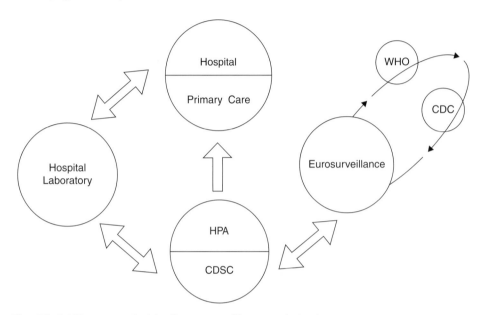

Fig. 18.1 UK communicable disease surveillance and alerting systems.

With this high index of suspicion, appropriate safety measures can be implemented early. What should be done in terms of safety is to institute 'b' (barrier) precautions, which include immediate physical isolation of the child, restriction of the number of staff coming into contact with the child and institution of appropriate personal protective equipment (PPE) measures (see Chapter 17). The effect of correct application of these measures should be to reduce the risk to staff and other children. What is needed next is a safe transfer to an appropriate location.

During the assessment and initial treatment stages, appropriate life-saving treatment should be instituted as required, with due regard to personal safety. However, procedures requiring close contact should be carried out only with appropriate protection. Only necessary emergency procedures should be carried out until the child is located in a more secure environment. It is advisable to limit the transport of children for essential medical investigations only and for children to wear high-efficiency masks during transport. (Note, however, that to ensure high-quality diagnosis, especially for the first cases detected, radiographs should be performed in the radiology department rather than by mobile machine wherever possible.)

C – control

During the assessment, whoever is the team leader should allocate the task of 'safety controller' until the arrival of an infection control specialist. Tasks will consist of:

• Controlling access to the quarantined area

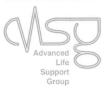

- Compliance with the correct PPE procedures
- Correct disposal of contaminated items
- Thorough cleaning and disinfection of the area and any equipment used during the transfer.

C – communication

Use a structured approach to communicate with the following:
- The consultant responsible for the care of the child
- The hospital manager on-call
- The infection control team in the trust
- The laboratories to inform them that 'high-risk' specimens will be sent
- The local medical microbiologist and chemical pathologist
- The local consultant in communicable disease control.

E – evaluation

The need to transfer the child to a secure environment should be discussed. In most cases this will be an intrahospital transfer. The competencies of accompanying staff will be dictated not only by their ability to ensure that infection transmission is minimised but also by the clinical needs of the child. Should it be imperative that an interhospital transfer be undertaken, appropriate arrangements should be made with the ambulance service. Helicopters and private transport should not be used.

P – preparation and packaging

Child and staff packaging must ensure that all reasonable measures are taken to ensure that any potential contamination of the staff, transfer equipment and the environment is reduced to a minimum.

T – transportation and handover

During the transfer, the team must remain alert to the possibility of a breach in the protective measures taken to limit contamination. Following handover, all equipment must be thoroughly cleaned and disinfected, disposable PPE equipment must be removed, taking care not to contaminate clean areas; this equipment must be disposed of in a safe manner. Finally, a record of all staff who have been in contact with the child should be made and passed to the infection control officer.

THE POTENTIALLY CONTAMINATED CHILD

Twenty-first century lifestyle depends on technology and chemicals. Each year over 49 million tonnes of chemicals are transported around the UK. The manufacture, storage and transportation of the most toxic chemicals are subject to stringent controls; however, accidents do happen. There is, of course, the constant worry about the deliberate release of chemicals into a public place.

Emergency services work together to develop contingency plans to respond rapidly to contain chemical incidents. The HPA is also involved in supporting the NHS in such emergency situations. These CBRN plans cover a wide range of possible scenarios: chemical, biological, radiological and nuclear. There are two main categories of chemical incident based on the speed of development of the incident:

1 Category I incident: in a category I incident (where the presentation is acute, and a chemical or toxic aetiology is most likely), decontamination is crucial in

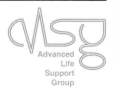

preventing secondary contamination. This will also be important in suspected overt deliberate release of a biological agent and where cases may have been exposed to, for example, unidentified powders or gases.

2 Category II incident: for a category II incident (where presentations may be more delayed and biological agents are rather more likely), the situation is more complicated because of the manner in which children might present. Although healthcare staff may be pre-warned of the arrival of cases of unusual illness, it is also possible that the healthcare staff will be the ones recognising the unusual nature of the presentation. As soon as there is any suspicion of an unusual aetiology, all staff should take precautions to protect themselves, primarily from biological agents (as above), although decontamination might once again be appropriate if the clinical picture is suggestive of chemical exposure.

> Only clean, or decontaminated, casualties will be transported to hospital by ambulance.

One of the primary functions of the emergency services' response to an acute chemical (category I) incident is decontaminating those who are likely to have been contaminated. This involves the difficult task of preventing the public from leaving the scene of the incident without decontamination.

Despite their best efforts, some people escape the cordon, only to present themselves at hospital later. It is worth noting that many of the casualties, following the 1994 Tokyo nerve agent (Sarin gas) attack, were contaminated at the receiving hospitals. This is because no early decontamination took place at the scene, no PPE was worn in the initial stages and no control was placed on contaminated members of the general public; therefore, self-referrals added to the problem, a situation that is likely to be the case within the UK. On entry to the warm hospital environment, the contaminated casualties began to 'off gas', thus contaminating those medical professionals attempting to save their lives.

Decontamination of self-referrals is a hospital NHS trust responsibility. There is likely to be some prior warning that casualties will arrive in an emergency department and cases should have been decontaminated before transfer to hospital. If this has not been performed then it should be done immediately on arrival at hospital. Specialist decontamination techniques are taught on training courses such as HAZIMMS (hazardous materials incident medical management and support).

Types of contamination

The modes of chemical contamination (Table 18.2) are similar to those described in Table 18.3.

Table 18.2 Modes of chemical contamination

Transmission route	Involves
Direct contact	Primary contamination
Droplets	Primary contamination
Airborne	Primary contamination
Indirect contact	Secondary contamination, contamination by another person

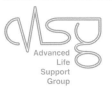

Table 18.3 Details of several modes of transmission of infection

Transmission route	Involves
Direct contact	Direct transmission of body fluids
Indirect contact	Indirect transmission of body fluids via an intermediate agent: personnel, equipment, hard surfaces
Airborne	Aerosol droplet spread (not usually >1m)
Indirect contact	Small particles ($\leq 5\,\mu m$) or infected dust may travel long distances depending on airflows

There are two main types of exposure to a contaminant:

1 Primary contamination: exposure where the contaminated person was in the vicinity of the agent when it was released. Any person who has suffered primary contamination must be thoroughly decontaminated.

2 Secondary contamination: exposure where a person has come into contact with an individual who has suffered primary exposure before decontamination.

Transfer

Children with significant injuries warranting transfer to a tertiary centre will almost certainly have been brought to the hospital by the ambulance service, whose members will have decontaminated them at scene. Therefore, the issue of the interhospital transfer of a chemically contaminated child should not arise. However, some children with minor injuries that still warrant admission may be brought in independently by their parents; these children, if identified as potentially contaminated, must be decontaminated outside the Emergency Department before admission and transfer to a ward.

SUMMARY

It is important to distinguish between infectious and chemically contaminated children. Applying a structured approach to safety throughout using the ACCEPT approach is vitally important to prevent the transmission of infectious diseases to healthcare workers and other children. Alert staff, who make the best use of barrier precautions, will help to prevent the spread of infectious diseases during the transfer process. The chemically contaminated child must be decontaminated before any transfer.

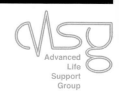

CHAPTER 19

Governance, legal and insurance issues

LEARNING OBJECTIVES

In this chapter you will learn about:

- An overview of clinical governance
- The need to be aware of the legal issues surrounding transfers and retrievals
- The difference between vicarious liability and accident insurance

---

INTRODUCTION

The introduction of a formal, structured approach to clinical governance in 1988 has led some to believe that it is a relatively new concept. In fact, the broad principles have been applied by healthcare professionals since the inception of the NHS in the 1940s. Its application applies to all staff working in health care. In this chapter we provide a brief overview of the approach to the delivery of good clinical governance.

In addition to the competencies to deliver good clinical care, hospital staff need a clear understanding of the legal framework within which they operate for their own, the patients' and the organisation's benefit. Medicolegal issues are by nature both varied and complex. This chapter focuses only on the key legal issues that should be considered when undertaking interhospital transport. This is by no means definitive and there is no substitute for accessing local expert advice for specific issues, as this text cannot offer definitive guidance.

The possibility of being injured in an accident when undertaking interhospital transfers is only too real. The detail of insurance cover available to transport staff can be extremely difficult to ascertain. In the final part of this chapter we suggest a model of cover that might be considered in your trust.

GOVERNANCE

Clinical governance was formalised out of the need for accountability of the safe delivery of health services. At its inception in 1998 it was defined in the consultation document *A First Class Service: Quality in the new NHS* (Department of Health 1998) as:

Paediatric and Neonatal Safe Transfer and Retrieval: The Practical Approach, Edited by Steve Byrne, Steve Fisher, Peter-Marc Fortune, Cassie Lawn and Sue Wieteska. © 2008 Blackwell Publishing, ISBN: 978-1-4051-6919-6.

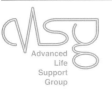

A framework through which NHS organisations are accountable for continuously improving the quality of their services and safeguarding high standards of care by creating an environment in which excellence in clinical care will flourish.

A common model used to illustrate the principal components of clinical governance is the seven pillars of excellence supported by five foundation stones as shown in Figure 19.1.

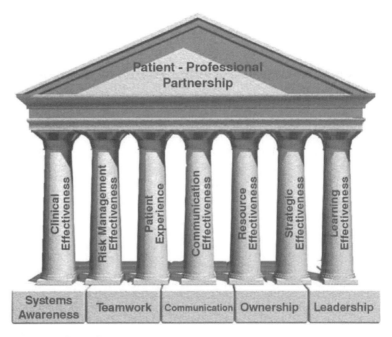

Fig. 19.1 Seven pillars of governance.

The key government bodies associated with this process have changed their titles several times in recent years. Currently, they comprise the National Institute for Health and Clinical Excellence (NICE), the Healthcare Commission (IICC) and the Clinical Governance Support Team (CGST). They are involved in regulation and facilitation of delivery of good clinical governance in partnership with the NHS workforce. It should not be forgotten that it is the responsibility of all employees within the NHS, both clinical and non-clinical, to ensure the delivery of a safe, high-quality service. In our area of interest, the planning and delivery of a children's transport service will require a risk assessment, proactive planning and constant audit with benchmarking to ensure service improvement.

For each of these areas, or 'pillars', there are specific standards against which trusts are judged and held accountable. For instance, safety issues (see Chapter 17) are assessed against current health and safety legislation and other appropriate guidance and legislation. Governance ensures that probity, patient safety, quality assurance and quality improvement are core components of all healthcare organisational activities. This is achieved through the culture of an organisation in which working practices demonstrate both managerial and clinical leadership, and accountability.

TRANSPORT LEAD PERSONNEL

An identified medical and nursing lead clinician must always be identified with responsibility for directing the transport service. This role would include: guideline approval, overseeing staff training, ensuring that equipment is fit for purpose and setting service level agreements. The director or an appropriate identified deputy must be contactable at all times for professional guidance on any problems. This individual is responsible for providing an overall clinical governance lead for the service.

STAFF TRAINING

Trusts with a designated transport service and identified staff should provide specific transport training. Selected staff must be able to demonstrate not only their competence and experience in children's intensive care, but also their ability to apply this in the transport setting. Retrieval training must prepare staff to manage the logistical aspects of any transport efficiently and safely and prepare, use and troubleshoot all of the equipment. They should also be familiar with all the relevant documentation and guidelines. Competency assessment should be used for both medical and nursing staff. This will require documentation for both trainer and trainee to sign and will serve as a record that training has been undertaken and completed satisfactorily.

VICARIOUS LIABILITY

We all have a duty of care to our patients. Organisationally, the NHS has a duty to ensure quality in the health care that it delivers. It passes most of that duty on to local healthcare trusts. Within a trust the chief executive carries responsibility for the maintenance of standards within the trust. Theoretically, that person is ultimately responsible for the actions and omissions of all staff employed by the trust. This responsibility is known as vicarious liability.

The chief executive and his or her team will seek to ensure appropriate professional development for all clinical staff in order to ensure quality. Provided that staff act reasonably, and within their competence, the chief executive will honour the responsibility for vicarious liability for all work undertaken on behalf of the trust, wherever that work takes place. This includes work undertaken while transferring a patient to or from another hospital. It is important to note that, if staff are judged to have acted unreasonably, and outside their competence or normal scope of practice, the trust may not consider itself responsible for the effects of the acts and omissions of these staff. The staff themselves may find themselves liable.

NEGLIGENCE

When there is a perception, from any quarter, that things have gone wrong, there may be allegations of negligence. Legal proof of negligence requires fulfilment of specific criteria. To prove a case of negligence the following must be established:
- A duty of care existed
- There was a failure of that duty of care
- The patient suffered some harm
- A chain of causation can be demonstrated that links all three of the above.

Unless all the above criteria are established, negligence cannot be proved. A failure to document the care of a patient thoroughly, particularly if there is an untoward event, may seriously harm your defence!

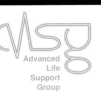

RECORD KEEPING

A contemporaneous record of all the key events of a transfer episode should be made. This should start with the details of the initial telephone call requesting transfer and cover the time through to the handover to the receiving hospital staff, or the decision not to transfer. All communications, face to face or via telephone, should be documented. Independent or regional transport services, which are not based at the receiving intensive care unit, will need to keep their own copies of the transport record and also make copies, available at the point of handover to the receiving unit. These copies should be filed in the child's hospital inpatient record. These records must be stored by both the hospital and the transport service, in this instance, for the recommended statutory period (currently 25 years for children).

In addition to written documentation, some transport services also use a telephone recording system. This records all calls initiated or received through the identified telephone lines/extensions. All callers must be made aware of the recording system, either with a pre-recorded message before the call is answered or by the staff member answering the call. Likewise, if a conference calling facility is used, each additional individual joining the call should be introduced to ensure that all parties are aware of who is participating in the conversation. These telephone recordings must be downloaded and stored in the same way as documented records, for the same statutory period.

ACCOUNTABILITY

The boundaries of clinical responsibilities

Simply put, the referring consultant in charge of the child's care will remain responsible for that care until the transfer team have received handover, assessed the patient and formally accepted the child into their care. Thereafter, the responsibility for clinical care ultimately rests with the consultant in charge of the team undertaking the transfer. However, the boundaries are often blurred; the transfer team will usually recommend a management plan to be followed after their arrival. This would be considered expert advice. Assuming that the advice is followed, the lead consultant of the transfer team will then take some responsibility for the consequences of their advice being followed. Where advice is not followed and a poor outcome occurs, it will be for the local team to explain why they took an alternative course (appropriately or otherwise). It may also be required that the transport team be required to demonstrate that they gave appropriate advice. In the absence of such evidence an expert team might be criticised for not providing appropriate guidance.

There may be a particularly difficult period during stabilisation, preparation and packaging where a junior grade transport doctor is working under the scrutiny of a local consultant. Again clear communication and accurate documentation are key. Usually the local team will be very supportive and it is advisable for transport teams to use all available resources. They should request senior local support as appropriate. For example, a paediatric middle grade transport doctor should request the help of a consultant anaesthetist from the referring hospital if an intubation were expected to be difficult.

The boundaries of clinical responsibility become particularly blurred when dealing with specialist referrals. For example, a referring hospital may receive advice from the specialist centre that may indicate a course of treatment to be started before transfer. The question arises as to who is responsible for the care of the patient before transfer. Is it the referring medical team or the receiving specialist medical team that is offering advice? A simple example may be a head-injured patient in one hospital being referred to a neuroscience centre at another hospital; the neuroscience hospital recommends 500 ml 20% mannitol, but the referring hospital declines to administer this drug and there is a subsequent legal argument as to who was responsible for the poor outcome of the patient. There is currently no legislation as to who takes majority accountability during these periods of joint care.

When the situation requires the referring hospital to undertake the interhospital transfer, it is not uncommon for the medical or surgical teams to ask the anaesthetic service to manage the transfer. The lines of responsibility will alter between teams in the same way as would occur using an external transfer service for specialist referrals. Therefore the local team, the anaesthetic team and the receiving (specialist) centre will all assume some part of the responsibility of care. The structured approach described in this manual should therefore be followed, especially with regard to handover and documentation that may be minimal or even omitted in these circumstances.

Negligence claims in respect of morbidity and mortality will have to prove the likely origin (time and place) of the act or omission that resulted in injury in order to apportion blame correctly. In other words, a receiving hospital cannot be held responsible for an act or omission that occurred before it had been contacted and will not assume the greater part of the responsibility until the patient is fully handed over and accepted into their team's care.

DEATH DURING TRANSPORT

The transport consultant should always be involved in any decision to move a child whom the transport clinicians consider to be at a high risk of dying. Normally there should be a discussion at consultant level by the referring and transport team to ensure that it is appropriate to move the child. The situation and risks should be explained to the parents and they should be given an opportunity both to question the decisions taken and to refuse permission to transfer where appropriate. Telephone conference call facilities may enable all parties to be simultaneously involved in the discussion, enhancing clarity and transparency. These discussions and the decision taken must be thoroughly documented in the clinical notes. If any person disagrees with the chosen course this should be documented, together with their reasons for disagreeing where possible.

Should the child die during transfer, the exact location of the death will determine which coroner oversees the case. This may alter the hospital to which you take the child. If it is an international ground transfer the exact location determines jurisdiction. However, if it is an air transfer, the pilot must be notified because the designation of the airspace and nationality of the airline may affect the decision of where to land under international aviation law.

DO NOT ATTEMPT RESUSCITATION ORDERS

In exceptional circumstances the transport team may be requested to transport a child with a do not attempt resuscitation (DNAR) order. This decision and DNAR order must be made jointly among the referring, receiving and transport staff at consultant level, and must include the consent of the parents. This decision, including details of any appropriate interventions, must be documented and

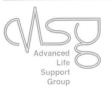

signed in both the clinical notes of the referring hospital and the transport notes.

DISABILITY AND DISABLEMENT ENTITLEMENT/INSURANCE COVER

All NHS staff are entitled to benefit from the NHS Injury Benefits Scheme. There is no qualifying period: everyone is covered from the day that they join the NHS. The scheme is not part of the NHS Pension Scheme; it is governed by different rules. It covers all NHS employees and general practitioners, whether or not they are members of the NHS Pension Scheme.

The NHS Injury Benefits Scheme provides a spectrum of benefits to the employee, in relation to temporary or permanent inability to work, up to and including death. In essence, the benefits are based on the present salary of the employee, years of service and, in the case of death, any dependants. These benefits are subject to a form of means test and may be curtailed if other compensation for the injury or benefits from other sources is being paid out. NHS trusts do subscribe to what is commonly known as employer's liability insurance schemes.

The NHS Litigation Authority is the insurance broker for NHS trusts. Details of benefits that may be obtained from this scheme are not clear: What is clear is that some form of negligence on the part of the employer may have to be proved, and the maximum compensation is rather limited.

As a result of the formation of the NHS Litigation Authority, NHS trusts are technically no longer permitted to enrol their staff in personal accident insurance schemes. Following this ruling, the Intensive Care Society (ICS, UK) arranged personal accident insurance for its members. This comprehensive insurance package is available to all ICS members (nursing and allied professional staff may join the ICS at a reduced membership rate). Membership of the Association of Anaesthetists of Great Britain and Ireland (AAGBI) confers similar benefits. The common belief among nursing staff that membership of the Royal College of Nursing (RCN) confers automatic personal accident insurance benefits is wholly untrue: the RCN will, however, arrange introduction to an approved insurance broker.

It is now widely accepted that a recognised transport service, whether a large-scale independent service or a smaller service supported by staff from the paediatric intensive care unit (PICU) requires additional insurance cover. At the time of writing most paediatric transport services within the UK had additional cover in place. As this is not a frequently occurring requirement, a small number of brokers deal with these policies. When seeking cover it is important to give consideration specifically to the number of personnel and separate disciplines to be included. The schedule of benefits must specify the amount to be awarded in case of all levels of injury, including temporary total disablement and death. Any maximum limits for claim and any limitation on number of personnel within a team for benefit purposes should be explored. Loss of earnings may be difficult to establish satisfactorily because of the range of salaries among various team members, and the monthly variation caused by extra duty payments.

SUMMARY

Clinical governance provides a structure to drive towards high-quality medical care.

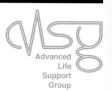

Transport is a particularly complex area. An understanding of the principles of vicarious liability and clinical negligence illustrates the importance of following the formal structures and approaches described in the ACCEPT approach. By following these principles, the patient should receive the best care possible and, should an untoward event occur, the clinical staff will receive all appropriate support through their trust and the legal system.

Staff undertaking interhospital transfers are advised that they should check that adequate financial arrangements are in place for themselves and their dependants in the event of an accident.

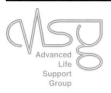

CHAPTER 20

Documentation

LEARNING OBJECTIVES

In this chapter you will learn about:
- The importance of transfer documentation
- The importance of a structured approach to documentation

INTRODUCTION

Throughout this manual reference has been made to the need for communication to be both structured and concise. During a transfer the majority of communications are undertaken verbally, either face to face or by telephone. It is important that the contents of key discussions are documented in the hospital notes, preferably on a custom-designed transfer proforma.

In Chapter 19 clinical governance was discussed as a methodology to measure and deliver good quality care. Good documentation underpins this process and is essential for any subsequent case reviews or audit. All of the Royal medical colleges and the Nursing and Midwifery Council (NMC) have issued statements about record keeping that are available to their members. Furthermore it is worth noting that all NHS records are public records under the terms of the Public Records Act 1958, and therefore may be accessed by anyone with appropriate permissions.

CLINICAL NOTES

Clinical notes are a legal record and a log of events. It is vital that they record not only the interventions and decisions that are taken, but also the basic clinical information that prompted these actions. Clinicians' handwriting is notorious for its illegibility; it should be considered that there is little point in using the pen to communicate if no one else can decipher what was written.

If a fact or event is not documented then, should you ever find yourself explaining your own actions in court, the event is generally regarded as not to have happened. Furthermore, if an entry is illegible, this not only represents a failure of communication but renders the entry inadmissible.

Paediatric and Neonatal Safe Transfer and Retrieval: The Practical Approach, Edited by Steve Byrne, Steve Fisher, Peter-Marc Fortune, Cassie Lawn and Sue Wieteska. © 2008 Blackwell Publishing, ISBN: 978-1-4051-6919-6.

CAUTION!

Anything you do, or say in the course of a child's treatment should be recorded in the clinical notes.

If you do not clearly document what you have said or done, it will harm your defence, if you later rely on your memory.

As with all documentation, each entry in the clinical notes should be dated, timed and signed. Furthermore the author's name, the General Medical Council (GMC) number if they are medical staff and status (for example, consultant paediatrician) should be clearly appended (Figure 20.1). It is good practice to note the location of the child, for example, 18/12/2006 12:23 St Elsewhere PICU Smith J. (Paediatric Registrar) bleep 2341 (GMC No: 1234567). This may be especially useful should you need to refer to the notes of a retrieval to explain your actions subsequently.

It is vitally important to record the date and time when events occurred, as well as the time that the entry was made. This is especially key when dealing with transfers, because the chronology of events and discussions may be crucial in an enquiry. If the pace of events and circumstances dictates that some entries must be made at a later time, this must be made clear; the notes should state that it is a 'non-contemporaneous' or 'retrospective' entry. They should include the time of the event referred to as well as the time that the entry was made.

As notes are written chronologically, there will inevitably be several sets of documentation covering:
- The referring hospital
- The transfer itself
- The receiving hospital.

Where possible it is preferable that the documentation reads as one continuous record. The referring hospital clinical notes should clearly summarise as shown in the box.

- The child's history
- The reasons for transfer
- Who has been involved in any discussions
- The assessments of the risks of transfer
- The consequent stabilisation procedures
- Ending up with a statement: 'child transferred to St Elsewhere Hospital, Ward 666'.

A suggested framework for documenting pre-transfer care is:
- Date and time of referral
- Name of referring clinician
- Name of referring consultant
- Diagnosis
- Clinical status of child
- Reason for transfer
- Actions agreed during referral process (and effect of these if any)
- Time of arrival and assessment of child

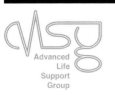

HMR 4 B (Code 090 0005)

....*Westminster*........ HOSPITAL

UNIT No. W 098 876

HISTORY SHEET

SURNAME (Block Letters) NICHOLLS

FIRST NAMES Harvey

DATE	CLINICAL NOTES (Each entry must be signed)

A.T.S by RMO

Risk assessment for transfer

to Leeds Paediatric Liver unit

26/05/2000
23:24
Ward 21
Bed 13
Wallace
Anaesthetics
Pager 3421

History as above.

Assessment:

Problem... 13 yr old Took 65 gm Paracetamol
36 hrs ago, Now developing acute liver failure

Actions:

Effect:

Next:

Potential risks:

A...   B...

C...   D...

Requires the following:

A...   B...

C...   D...

P.G. Wallace

GMC No: 1234567

Fig. 20.1 Clinical notes.

- Status of child on arrival
- Actions before transfer.

Intensive care personnel and anaesthetists may be called to assess a child who is to be transferred to another hospital for care. The notes should clearly indicate the reason for the request. In such cases the approach should include an assessment of transfer risk, and a logical evaluation leading to the conclusion about what staffing and equipment resources are required for this child. An example is shown in Figure 20.2.

Child's name.   DOB:
Problems:
1.
2.
3.
Request for transfer made by:
Reason for transfer:
Intended destination:
Summary clinical assessment:
Appropriate transfer? YES / NO
If Yes – Actions required before transfer / If No reason for declining request:

Names and designations of transport team (if appropriate)
Transfer approved by ....(Name of consultant)

Fig. 20.2 Assessment of request for transfer.

TRANSFER FORMS

Some form of transfer documentation, which provides a summary of care, must be completed during and after the transfer.

Just as both hospitals will have a unique record number for each child, the ambulance service will issue a unique record number for each ambulance journey – the incident number. This number should be recorded on the transfer form to facilitate audit and investigation of adverse incidents.

Copies of the transfer form should be filed in the referring hospital's notes, the receiving hospital's notes and a central point for audit. Part of a sample transfer form is shown in Appendix E.

SUMMARY

Effective oral and written communication is an essential part of the transfer process. All communication must be structured, clear and concise. Key oral communications should be recorded in the clinical notes.

The documentation of the events surrounding a transfer is important not only for clinical audit, but also for your own protection should litigation arise.

The last page of the referring hospital's notes, the transfer form and the first pages of the receiving hospital's notes should read as a seamless progression of events. The reader should be able to follow the thought processes that guided the chain of events bringing about the transfer of the critically ill child. The notes should also reflect the high standard of care and communication during this difficult time.

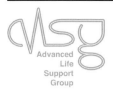

PART VI
Appendices

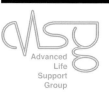

APPENDIX A

Intensive care levels: classification of ICU patient dependency

This issue is classified by paediatric intensive care unit (PICU) and neonatal ICU (NICU) in slightly different ways.

- In a PICU the description is patient based but may be applied to describe a unit. For example, a level 1 critical care area, for children needing greater attention than can be provided on the ward, is generally classed as a high dependency unit (HDU). Many district general hospitals (DGHs) will be able to provide level 2 care for a period of time without difficulty. However, level 3 and 4 care is generally delivered only by specialised PICUs.
- In NICU the description applies to the capabilities of the NICU itself. Similar to above some DGHs will be able to provide level 1 care for a period of time but would be expected to manage level 2 patients only for short periods. These children are transferred to specialist NICU centres.

	PICU	NICU
Level 1	High dependency care requiring nurse: patient ratio 0.5:1	Units that provide special care but do not aim to provide continuing high dependency or intensive care. This category includes units with or without resident medical staff
Level 2	A child requiring continuous nursing supervision who is usually intubated and ventilated. Also the unstable non-intubated child, e.g. a child who has recently been extubated. Nurse:patient ratio 1:1	Units that provide high dependency care and some short-term intensive care as agreed within their network
Level 3	A child requiring intensive supervision at all times, who needs additional complex therapeutic procedures and nursing. For example, unstable ventilated children on vasoactive drugs, inotropic support or multiple organ failure. Level 2 children in a cubicle. Nurse:patient ratio 1.5:1	Units that provide the whole range of medical neonatal care but not necessarily all specialist services such as neonatal surgery

Continued

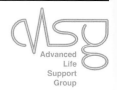

	PICU	NICU
Level 4	A child requiring the most intensive interventions such as level 3 patients nursed in a cubicle and children requiring renal replacement therapy. Nurse:patient ratio 2:1	
Level 5	This is a non-standardised definition for a child requiring intensive treatment modalities available only in quaternary centres. In practice this specifically refers to children requiring ECMO therapy. Nurse:patient ratio may be >2:1	

ECMO, extracorporeal membrane oxygenation; ICU, intensive care unit; NICU, neonatal ICU; PICU, paediatric ICU.

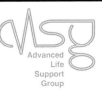

APPENDIX B

The PaNSTaR transfer master: a summary of ACCEPT

ASSESSMENT	*'What else would you like to know?'*
	1 Identifies key issues: 　What is wrong 　What do you need 2 Attempts structured approach to assessment 3 Considers most appropriate placement of patient
CONTROL	*'What actions would you undertake?'*
	1 Identify transport team and leader 2 Identify tasks – equipment/staff 3 Identify tasks – pre-transport advice 4 Identify tasks – liaise with units/ambulance 5 Ensure tasks allocated and documented
COMMUNICATION	*'To whom and how would you communicate this?'*
	1 Considers structure of communication 2 Considers content of communication: 　Who you are 　What is needed – from the listener 　What the patient's basic details are 　What the problem is 　What has been done 　What the response was 　What is needed 3 Are key parties communicated with?
EVALUATION	*'What further decisions are now required?'*
	1 Establishes urgency of transfer 2 Establishes appropriateness of transfer 3 Considers mode of transfer

PREPARATION	*'What would you do before transferring the patient?'*
PACKAGING PRE-DEPARTURE CHECKS	1 Actions on arrival 2 Undertakes handover 3 Optimises patient's condition – ABC, etc. 4 Communication with family 5 Secures equipment to patient 6 Prepares trolley, incubator and ambulance 7 Packages patient 8 Pre-departure checks

TRANSPORTATION	*'What are the important aspects for the return journey?'*
	1 Ensures equipment securely loaded 2 Monitoring and documentation 3 Appropriate road speed 4 Logical approach to troubleshooting 5 Appropriate handover

Advanced
Life
Support
Group

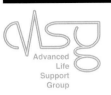
Advanced
Life
Support
Group

APPENDIX C

Transfer aide-memoire

AIRWAY

Item	Notes
Guedel size (guide)	Centre of mouth to angle of jaw
Nasopharyngeal airway (guide)	Diameter as ET tube (size of the child's little finger) Length – tip of the nose to the tragus of the ear
Endotracheal (ET) tube approximate size	**Preterm**

Preterm

Weight	Internal diameter (mm)	Length at lips
<1.0 kg	2.5	5.5–6.5
1–3 kg	3.0	7–8.5
>3 kg	3.5	8.5–9

Infants and children

Age	Internal diameter (mm)
<9 months	3.5
>1 year	(Age/4) + 4

Item	Notes
ET tube approximate length (cm) (from 1 year of age)	Oral: (Age/2) + 12 Nasal: (Age/2) + 15
Suction catheter for ET tube	French gauge is numerically twice the internal diameter in millimetres
Laryngoscopes suitable for age	Include straight blade for children up to 5 years

BREATHING

Item	Notes
Self-inflating bags with reservoir	240 ml if preterm neonate – check that valve works 500 ml for infants and neonates – check that valve works 1600 ml for child and older child
Mask size to fit child	Infants circular 0/1, 1, 2 Child anatomical 2, 3 Adolescent 4, 5
End-tidal CO_2 intubated patients Paediatric sized chest tubes	To fit between ribs

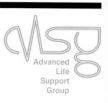

CIRCULATION

Formula to calculate weight in kg 1–10 years = 2 (Age + 4).

Item	Notes
Blood pressure cuffs	The width of the cuff should be more than 80% of length of upper arm/leg and the bladder more than 40% of the arm's circumference
Blood pressure	Guideline minimum mean blood pressure by age:
	Preterm < 28 days old
	Mean BP (mmHg) ≥ Gestational age (weeks)
	Infants and children
	Neonate 40 mmHg
	3 months 45 mmHg
	6 months–3 years 50 mmHg
	7–10 years 60 mmHg
	>12 years 70 mmHg
Defibrillation	**VF and pulseless VF**
Pre-departure check: check what	4 J/kg for all shocks
your machine will deliver	**Synchronised cardioversion**
	First shock 1 J/kg
	Second shock 2 J/kg
	Continue at 2 J/kg for subsequent shocks
Bolus adrenaline (epinephrine)	10 mcg/kg
	(0.1 ml/kg of 1 in 10 000 strength)
	or the dose is given via ET tube
Fluid bolus	20 ml/kg (10 ml/kg in trauma with possible head injury)
Inotrope infusions	**Dopamine/Dobutamine**
(It is preferable to use the	15 mg/kg in 50 ml 0.9% saline will give 5 mcg/kg
concentrations used by your local	per min if run at 1 ml/h
tertiary unit)	**Adrenaline/Noradrenaline**
	0.3 mg/kg in 50 ml 0.9% saline will give 0.1 mcg/kg
	per min if run at 1 ml/h
Peripheral intravenous catheters	All sizes should be available: 14 G (brown) 16 G (grey); 18 G (green); 20 G (pink); 22 G (blue); 24 G (yellow); 26 G (white). Always site largest possible for transfer
Intraosseous access	Anterior (medial) surface of tibia (ensure can access easily) 2–3 cm below tibial tuberosity
Central venous catheters	4, 5 and 7 Fr, 5–20 cm, two to three lumina. Appropriate size and length to be specified by experienced operator
Urinary catheter	Neonate nasogastric tube 5 Fr/6 Fr
	Infant 6–8 Fr Foley with balloon
	1–12 years 6–8 Fr Foley with balloon
	Adolescent 8–14 Fr Foley with balloon

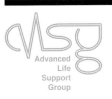

DISABILITY

Item	Notes
Printed coma scale	Child/Adult versions should be available
Cerebral perfusion pressure (CPP)	CPP = MAP − ICP
	[MAP = (Systolic + 2 × Diastolic)/3]
Mannitol	Dose is 0.25–0.5 g/kg (discuss indications with tertiary centre pre-transfer)
Glucose meter and 10% glucose	Check glucose; if stix test <3 mmol/l give 10% dextrose as bolus dose of 5 ml/kg

ICP, intracranial pressure; MAP, mean arterial pressure.

DRUGS

Item	Notes
Paediatric/Neonatal arrest box	Standardised box for hospital
Intubation drugs	Choose for familiarity and clinical indications, pre-calculate doses before starting transfer
Seizure drugs	Intravenous lorazepam 100 mcg/kg; can be repeated
	Diazepam rectally 0.5 mg/kg
	Phenytoin 18 mg/kg

EXPOSURE

- Pre-warm the ambulance
- Cover the head, wrap carefully
- Paracetamol/ibuprofen doses pre-calculated in case of fever.

WHY TREAT CHILDREN DIFFERENTLY?

Endotracheal tube

Oral length (cm)	Internal diameter (mm)
18–21	7.5–8.0
18	7.0
17	6.5
16	6.0
15	5.5
14	5.0
13	4.5
12	4.0
	3.5
10	3.0–3.5

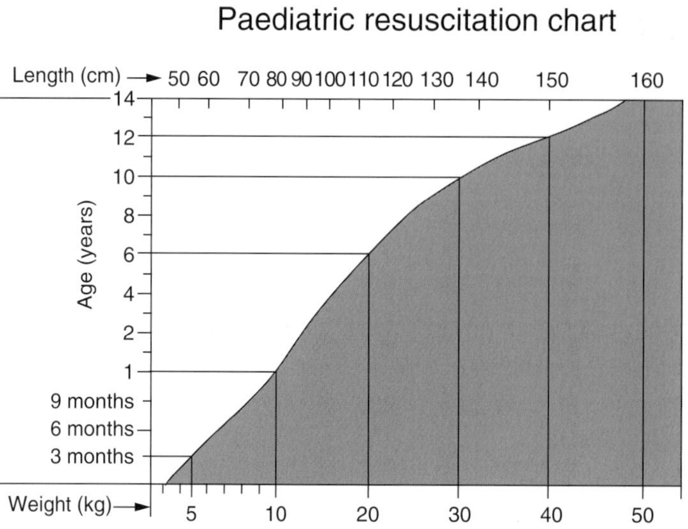

Paediatric resuscitation chart

Length (cm) → 50 60 70 80 90 100 110 120 130 140 150 160

Age (years) / Weight (kg) →

	5	10	20	30	40	50
Adrenaline/Epinephrine						
mL of 1 in 10 000 IV/IO	0.5	1	2	3	4	5
mL of 1 in 1000 ET	0.5	1	2	3	4	5
mL of 1 in 10 000 deep IM – *in anaphylaxis*	0.5	1	-	-	-	-
mL of 1 in 1000 deep IM – *in anaphylaxis*	-	0.1	0.2	0.3	0.4	0.5
Atropine [1]						
mL of 100 µg/mL IV/IO	1	2	4	6	8	10
mL of 600 µg/mL IV/IO	-	0.3	0.7	1	1.3	1.7
Amiodarone [2] *dilute in 5% glucose* for infusion						
mL of 30 mg/mL (pre-filled) IV/IO	0.8	1.5	3.5	5	6.5	8.5
mL of 50 mg/mL (concentrated) IV/IO	0.5	1	2	3	4	5
Bicarbonate [3]						
mmol IV/IO	5	10	20	30	40	50
Calcium chloride [4]						
mL of 10% IV/IO	0.5	1	2	3	4	5
DC Defibrillation [5]						
Joules	20	40	60	120	150	150
Initial DC Cardioversion [6]						
Joules	5	5	10	15	20	25
Fluid bolus [7]– *halve in uncontrolled bleeding*						
mL IV/IO	100	200	400	600	800	1000
Glucose						
mL of 10% IV/IO	25	50	100	150	200	250
Lorazepam						
mL of 4 mg *diluted* to 4 mL in 0.9% saline IV/IO	0.5	1	2	3	4	4
mL of 4 mg/mL *neat IV/IO*	-	-	0.5	0.75	1	1
Diazepam						
mg PR	2.5	5	10	10	10	10
Midazolam [8]						
mL of 10 mg/mL buccal	-	0.5	0.75	1	1	1
Naloxone						
mL of 400µg/mL IM – *if no vascular access*	1	-	-	-	-	-
mL of 400µg/mL IV/IO	0.125	0.25	0.5	0.75	1	1.25

[1] Atropine 100 µg/mL can be prepared by diluting 1 mg to 10 mL (or 600 µg to 6 mL) in 0.9% saline.
[2] Amiodarone is given as a bolus in cardiac arrest. Otherwise give as an infusion over 30 minutes, diluted with 5% dextrose to a total volume of 1-2 mL/kg.
[3] Bicarbonate 8.4% has 1 mmol/mL, 4.2% has 0.5 mmol/mL and 1.26% has 0.15 mmol/mL. Do not use undiluted 8.4% in infants.
[4] Note that 1 mL of calcium chloride 10% is equivalent to 3 mL of calcium gluconate 10% or 0.75 mL of calcium chloride 13.4%. Only use in documented hypocalcemia, hyperkalemia, hypermagnesemia and calcium channel blocker overdose. Give as a bolus when indicated in cardiac arrest or otherwise slowly over 5-10 minutes and consider repeating if necessary.
[5] Use 4 J/kg for initial or repeated shocks with either biphasic or monophasic defibrillator.
[6] Cardiovert in SVT with shock (synchronous). If synchronous fails in SVT, use asynchronous.
[7] If *uncontrolled bleeding* is suspected, use 10 mL/kg rather than 20 mL/kg as a fluid bolus, while emergency interventions to stop the bleeding are being implemented. Repeat after re-assessment, if necessary. This approach is similar to 'permissive hypotension', 'delayed fluids' or 'deliberate under-resuscitation' in adults.
[8] An equivalent dose of the *intravenous* (but not the *oral*) may be used if the *buccal* preparation is not available.

Fig. C.1 Oakley Chart.

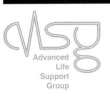

APPENDIX D

Checklists

CORE EQUIPMENT (CHECK PRE-DEPARTURE FROM BASE AND REFERRAL HOSPITAL)

Incubator/Pod	Syringe drivers	Fridge drugs/Prostin
Baby pod cover	Monitor	Oxygen calculation
Prepacked transport kit 1	Monitor mains lead	Oxygen cylinders
Prepacked transport kit 2	Monitor ambulance lead	Mobile phone
Vacuum mat	BP cuff	ABG analyser
Transfer form	End-tidal CO_2	ABG analyser consumables

ADDITIONAL EQUIPMENT

	iNO calculation	Sharps bin
Air cylinders	iNO cylinders	Suction
Air cylinder head	iNO delivery system	Defibrillator
Transwarmer mattress	Croup tubes	Long haul battery
Flight bag	Laryngeal masks	

OUTWARD JOURNEY

Connect power	Monitor	Incubator	Syringe drivers

ARRIVAL AT REFERRING CENTRE

Connect power	Monitor	Incubator	Syringe drivers

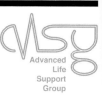

PRE-DEPARTURE CHECKLIST

Airway/Breathing	Chest X-ray checked
	ABG post-placement on transport ventilator
	Humidivent/viral filter
	End-tidal CO_2
	Oxygen/air available in sufficient quantity
	Airway/drug bag
	AmbuBag
	Secondary bagging oxygen
Circulation	Appropriate BP/circulation monitoring
Drugs/fluids	Sufficient and working intravenous access
	Sedation, analgesia, paralysis
Sedation	Appropriate analgesia/sedation/paralysis
Other	Nasogastric tube free drainage
	Chest drains on Heimlich valve
	Equipment packed (see minimum equipment list above)
Paperwork/communication	Transport consultant informed and plan agreed
	Maternal blood if surgical neonate
	Receiving unit contacted
	ECMO consent
	Chest X-ray, CT scans and notes copied

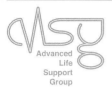

Advanced
Life
Support
Group

APPENDIX E

Generic referral form

ICU: {...}   Contact Numbers   Mobile:{...}

EXTERNAL REFERRAL FORM

Referral Number	Ambulance Booking Number

Referral Details

Referral call taken by		Date	
Name of referring doctor	Telephone:		Bleep:
Name of referring consultant:	Mobile:		Referring consultant aware? Present / Yes / No

Child's details

Child's name		Male/Female/Unassigned
Weight: Kg	Date of Birth:	Gestation: /40 (Corrected) age:

Child's Location

Hospital:	Ward/Unit:	Ward Telephone:

Provisional diagnosis

Timeline

Referral Call	
Accepted	
Ambulance booked	
Ambulance arrive	
Base departure	
Referring centre Arrival	
Departure	
Return to base	

Clinical Details

Call returned by	Time
Date and time of admission to referring hospital	
History	

Advice given

Name of clinician at referring centre receiving advice:	Agreed with referrer	Actioned on arrival
1.	1 ☐	1 ☐
2.	2 ☐	2 ☐
3.	3 ☐	3 ☐
4.	4 ☐	4 ☐
5.	5 ☐	5 ☐

	Reason for non-compliance with advice? (If applicable - Continue in comments section if needed)
Signed	

Physiology on referral (Please also document compliance with advice on front page)

asg
Advanced
Life
Support
Group

ICU: {...}   Contact Numbers   **Mobile:{...}**

Resp rate /min	**Ventilation status**			**Access**	
O₂ Sats %	ETT	Size mm	Length cm	Number of peripheral lines:	
Recession? Yes / No	Facemask		% l/min	Central line	Yes / No
FiO₂	Nasal cannula		l/min	Arterial line	Yes / No
Heart rate /min	Headbox O₂		%	Interosseous Line	Yes / No
CRT s	GCS	E	M	V	**Resuscitation volume**	
BP /	Pupils reactive?		Yes / No	Total given:	ml
CVP cmH₂O	Pupils equal?		Yes / No	Over how long?	min

Results

Blood gas			**Laboratory**	
Time:	Time:	Time:	Time:	
Art/Cap/Venous	Art/Cap/Venous	Art/Cap/Venous	Hb	Na⁺
pH	pH	pH	WCC	K⁺
pCO₂	pCO₂	pCO₂	Plates	Ca²⁺
pO₂	pO₂	pO₂	CRP	Glucose
HCO₃	HCO₃	HCO₃	Lactate	Urea
BXS	BXS	BXS	INR	Creatinine
Lactate	Lactate	Lactate		

Other relevant results:

Anaesthetic Assessment

Anaesthetist Name:	Grade:	Time of assessment

Assessment made

Assessment

Referral discussed with:

(Consultant Name)

Accepted →	Bed _only_ offered		Bed & Retrieval offered	
Not Accepted →	Inappropriate referral	PICU full (No beds)	PICU (insufficient staff)	Other (please specify)

Transport team

Name	Grade

Pre-departure

Pre-departure Equipment Checklist Completed	Special Equipment Taken
Dr SIGN Nurse SIGN	

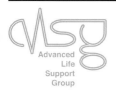

APPENDIX F

Transfer competences

The Paediatric Intensive Care Society is currently piloting a competency pro-
gramme for transfer of critically unwell children. It is anticipated that this will be
published concurrently with this manual (see www.ukpics.org).

Glossary

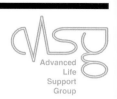

AAGBI	Association of Anaesthetists of Great Britain and Ireland
ABG	arterial blood gas
AC	alternating current
ARDS	acute respiratory distress syndrome
BIG	bone injection gun
BP	blood pressure
CAA	Civil Aviation Authority
CBRN	chemical, biological, radiological and nuclear
CCU	critical care unit
CDR Weekly	*Communicable Disease Report Weekly*
CDSC	Communicable Disease Surveillance Centre
CEN	European Committee for Standardisation
CGST	Clinical Governance Support Team
CLDP	chronic lung disease of prematurity
CNS	central nervous system
CO	cardiac output
CPAP	continual positive airway pressure
CPP	cerebral perfusion pressure
CT	computed tomography
CVP	central venous pressure
DC	direct current
DGH	district general hospital
DIC	diffuse intravascular coagulation
DKA	diabetic ketoacidosis
DNAR	do not attempt resuscitation
ECG	electrocardiogram
ECMO	extracorporeal membrane oxygenation
ENT	ear, nose and throat
ET	endotracheal
ETCO$_2$	end-tidal carbon dioxide
FiO_2	fraction of inspired oxygen
FRC	functional residual capacity
FS	fractional shortening
GMC	General Medical Council
HAZIMMS	hazardous materials incident medical management and support
HCC	Healthcare Commission
HDU	high dependency unit
HEMS	helicopter emergency medical services
HFJV	high-frequency jet ventilation
HFOV	high-frequency oscillatory ventilation
Hib	*Haemophilus influenzae* type b

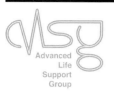

HME	heat moisture exchanger
HPA	health protection agency
HR	heart rate
ICP	intracranial pressure
ICS	Intensive Care Society
ICU	intensive care unit
IMV	intermittent mandatory ventilation
IVH	intraventricular haemorrhage
JRCALC	Joint Royal Colleges Ambulance Liaison Committee
MAP	mean arterial pressure
MAS	meconium aspiration syndrome
MOD	Ministry of Defence
MRI	magnetic resonance imaging
NEC	necrotising enterocolitis
NHS	National Health Service
NIBP	non-invasive blood pressure
NiCd	nickel–cadmium
NICE	National Institute for Health and Clinical Excellence
NICU	neonatal intensive care unit
NiMH	nickel metal hydride
NMC	Nursing and Midwifery Council
NO	nitric oxide
$PaCO_2$	partial pressure of CO_2 in alveoli
PaNSTaR	paediatric and neonatal safe transfer and retrieval
PaO_2	partial pressure of oxygen in alveoli
PAPR	powered air-purifying respirator
PCO_2	partial pressure of carbon dioxide
PEEP	positive end-expiratory pressure
PFC	persistent fetal circulation
PICANET	Paediatric Intensive Care Audit Network
PiCCO	a device that measures cardiac parameters using transpulmonary thermodilution techniques and arterial pulse contour analysis
PICU	paediatric intensive care unit
PIP	peak inspiratory pressure
PPE	personal protective equipment
PPHN	persistent pulmonary hypertension of the newborn
RAF	Royal Air Force
RCN	Royal College of Nursing
RDS	respiratory distress syndrome
RNAS	Royal Naval Air Rescue
RSV	respiratory syncytial virus
SaO_2	saturation of oxygen (arterial blood)
SARS	severe acute respiratory syndrome
SCBU	special care baby unit
SET	signal extraction technology
SLA	sealed lead acid
SpO_2	transcutaneous peripheral oxygen saturation
STaR	safe transfer and retrieval
SV	stroke volume
SVT	supraventricular tachycardia
$TcCO_2$	transcutaneous CO_2

TcO$_2$	transcutaneous O$_2$
TPN	total parenteral nutrition
UAC	umbilical arterial catheter
UVC	umbilical venous catheter
$\dot{V}/\dot{Q}$	ventilation/perfusion
VT	ventricular tachycardia

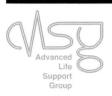

APPENDIX H

References and further information

Chapter 14

Joint Aviation Requirements. JAR OPS 3,005(D). Civil Aviation Authority.

Chapter 15

Association of Anaesthetists of Great Britain and Ireland. *Provision of Anaesthetic Services in Magnetic Resonance*. London: AAGBI, 2002. Available online at: www.aagbi.org/pdf/mri.pdf

Chen DW. Boy, 6, dies of skull injury during MRI; oxygen tank becomes fatal missile in hospital. *New York Times* July 31, 2001: p B1, 5.

Chapter 16

Advanced Life Support Group. *Advanced Paediatric Life Support: The practical approach*, 4th edn. Oxford: Blackwell Publishing Ltd, 2005.

Chapter 17

Becker LR, Zaloshnja E, Levick N, Li G, Miller TR. Relative risk of injury and death in ambulances and other emergency vehicles. *Accid Anal Prev* 2003;**35**:941–8.

Biggers WA Jr, Zachariah BS, Pepe PE. Emergency medical vehicle collisions in an urban system. *Prehospital Disaster Medicine* 1996;**11**:195–201.

Kahn CA, Pirrallo RG, Kuhn EM. Characteristics of fatal ambulance crashes in the united states: an 11-year retrospective analysis. *Prehospital Emergency Care* 2001;**5**:261–9.

Maguire BJ, Hunting KL, Smith GS, Levick NR. Occupational fatalities in emergency medical services: a hidden crisis. *Ann Emerg Med* 2002;**40**:625–32.

Chapter 19

Department of Health. *A First Class Service: Quality in the new NHS*. HSC 1998/113. London: DH, 1998.

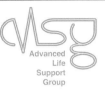

Index

Note: page numbers in *italics* refer to figures and boxes, those in **bold** refer to tables

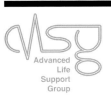

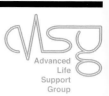

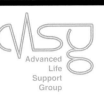

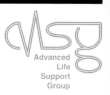

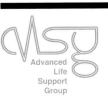

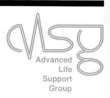

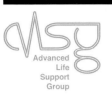

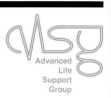

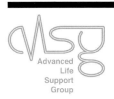

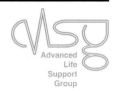

Other publications of interest

Acute Medical Emergencies:
The Practical Approach
Advanced Life Support Group
ISBN: 9780727914644
2000

Advanced Paediatric Life Support:
The Practical Approach
Fourth Edition
Advanced Life Support Group
ISBN: 9780727918475
2004

Major Incident Management System (MIMS)
Edited by Timothy Hodgetts (University of
Birmingham, Birmingham, UK) and Crispin Porter
(Frimley Park Hospital NHS Foundation
Trust, Frimley, UK)
ISBN: 9780727916143
2002

Major Incident Medical Management and
Support: The Practical Approach in the
Hospital (HMIMMS)
Advanced Life Support Group
ISBN: 9780727918680
2005

Major Incident Medical Management &
Support: The Practical Approach
At the Scene (MIMMS)
Second Edition
Advanced Life Support Group
ISBN: 9780727913913
2002

Pocket Guide to Teaching for Medical
Instructors
Second Edition
Edited by Ian Bullock (Lead Educator,
Resuscitation Council, UK), Mike Davis (Lead
Educator, ALSG, UK), *et al.*
ISBN: 9781405175692
2008

Pre-Hospital Paediatric Life Support:
The Practical Approach
Second Edition
Advanced Life Support Group
ISBN: 9780727918529
2005

Safe Transfer and Retrieval of Patients (STAR)
Second Edition
Advanced Life Support Group
ISBN: 9780727918550
2006

How to order these books
Phone:
UK Dial Free: 0800 243407
Overseas: +44 (0)1243 843294
US Toll Free: 877 762 2974
Canada Toll Free: 800 567 4797

Fax:
UK & Overseas: +44(0)1243 843296
US & Canada: 800 605 2665

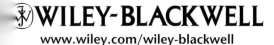

www.wiley.com/wiley-blackwell